Edgar Sheppard

Lectures On Madness In It's Medical, Legal, And Social Aspects

Edgar Sheppard

Lectures On Madness In It's Medical, Legal, And Social Aspects

ISBN/EAN: 9783741134449

Manufactured in Europe, USA, Canada, Australia, Japa

Cover: Foto ©Lupo / pixelio.de

Manufactured and distributed by brebook publishing software (www.brebook.com)

Edgar Sheppard

Lectures On Madness In It's Medical, Legal, And Social Aspects

LECTURES ON MADNESS

IN ITS

MEDICAL, LEGAL, AND SOCIAL ASPECTS

BY

EDGAR SHEPPARD, M.D.

MEMBER OF THE ROYAL COLLEGE OF PHYSICIANS, PROFESSOR OF PSYCHOLOGICAL MEDICINE
IN KING'S COLLEGE, LONDON, AND ONE OF THE MEDICAL SUPERINTENDENTS OF
THE MIDDLESEX COUNTY LUNATIC ASYLUM AT COLNEY HATCH.

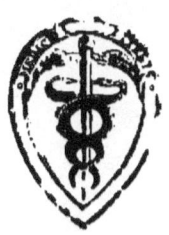

LONDON
J. & A. CHURCHILL, NEW BURLINGTON STREET
1873

TO

GEORGE JOHNSON, M.D., F.R.S.,
PROFESSOR OF MEDICINE IN KING'S COLLEGE, LONDON,

THE FRIEND AND FELLOW-STUDENT OF EARLIER,
THE TRIED FRIEND AND COLLEAGUE
OF LATER, YEARS,

I AFFECTIONATELY DEDICATE

THESE LECTURES.

CONTENTS.

LECTURE I.

Institution of Psychological Chair at King's College—Importance of Subject—Exciting Causes of Insanity—Its Prevalence—Predisposing Causes—Hereditary Nature of Insanity—Its Prevalence, and Ratio of Occurrence in the Two Sexes, and in Town and Country—Its Exciting Causes, Moral and Physical, and Difficulty of Defining the same—Importance of Early Treatment, and Difficulty thereof 1–31

LECTURE II.

Anatomy and Physiology of Nervous System—Pathological Changes as observed after Death—Classification of Insanity—Melancholia: Simple, Acute, Attonita—Treatment—Value of Turkish Bath—Artificial Feeding—Precaution against Suicide—Impulsive and Non-impulsive Acts of the Insane—Recurrent Character of Insanity 32–56

LECTURE III.

Mania—Transitoria or Acute Delirious—Illustrative Case—Diagnosis—Acute Mania—Illustrative Case—Prognosis—Treatment—Destructiveness—Simple Mania—Monomania (so-called)—Cunning of the Insane—*Folie Circulaire*—Recurrent Character of Insanity reiterated . . 57–86

LECTURE IV.

Moral Insanity (so-called)—Existence of Delusions not necessary to establish Madness—"Insane Temperament:" its Characteristics, and Frequent Association with Intellectuality—Illustrative Case of Moral Insanity—Tact and Management required in Treatment—Impulsive Insanity—Impulse not the First Evidence of Insanity—Case of Rev. J. S. Watson—Homicidal Impulse Masked by

Epilopsy in a Child—Case—Moral Insanity of later years, and its sequence—Dementia—Acute Primary Dementia—Chronic Primary Dementia—Secondary Dementia—Diagnosis of Acute Primary Dementia—Treatment—Attitudes, Untidiness, and Depraved Habits of Insane 87–112

LECTURE V.

Puerperal Insanity—Its Forms not Special or Peculiar to the Child-bearing State—Three Distinct Periods of Occurrence, and Three Forms—Illustrative Case of Puerperal Mania—Puerperal Melancholia—Frequent Association with Prolonged Lactation—Frequent Dislike by Patient of her Husband and Children—Suicidal Acts specially to be guarded against—Puerperal Dementia—Illustrative Case of Puerperal Cataleptoid Dementia—Relative Danger to Life and Reason of Puerperal Insanity—Treatment—Forced Separation of Patient from Friends 113–136

LECTURE VI.

General Paralysis of the Insane—A Tragedy in Three Acts: 1st Act, 2nd Act, 3rd Act—Epileptiform Seizures—Gradual Descent of the Physical and Moral Ladder—"Last Stage of All"—Deceptive Character of Improvement in Early Stages—Temporary Recoveries not Real—Sexual Indulgence—Nerve Power Speedily Exhausted thereby—Relative Frequency of General Paralysis in the Two Sexes—Average Duration of—Causation—Treatment—Pathological Changes 137–162

LECTURE VII.

Idiocy and Imbecility—Differential Characteristics—Moral Responsibility of the Fast "Not quite Right" Youths of Society—Difficulty of always determining the same—Plea of Insanity in those Cases—Criminal Responsibility in Homicidal Mania—Knowledge of Difference between Right and Wrong as a Test of Insanity—Impaired and Dominated Volition from Delusions and Hallucinations—Feigned Insanity—Hereditary Nature both of Crime and Insanity—Instructive Case of Malingering—Difficulty at times of Diagnosing the Real from the Pretended—Rules for Guidance—The "Non-restraint" System—The Excess to which it has been pushed in England—General Management of the Insane—Conclusion . . . 163–186

LECTURES ON MADNESS.

LECTURE I.

GENTLEMEN,

This is a new Chair, and I am a new Professor. The Council of King's College, following the example of other metropolitan schools, have in their wisdom thought fit to institute psychological teaching; and, honouring me as an old student of this place, and one largely familiar with insane life, they have charged me with the responsibility of leading you within the precincts of that domain, which is peopled alike by the wildest and the happiest, the tamest and most mournful, of mankind.

Now, you will naturally expect me to magnify the importance of that which I am about to bring under your notice, and which is the subject of my specialty. But really I have no desire to do anything of the kind. You will hardly expect me, at all events, to underrate it. For who can lightly estimate that which is of such stupendous interest, as embracing the higher part of man's nature? Whether we are descended (as some suppose) from simian conformations, or (as the majority of men think) there is an impassable gulf, which time and development can never bridge over, between those odoriferous travesties of humanity and ourselves, it is equally certain that the breath of life has been breathed into us by Omnipotence, and we are supposed, in contradistinction from all other living creatures, to be bound for a larger and more enduring destiny beyond the confines of this world.

To have this higher part, then, deranged, " out of gear," and not perfectly *d'accord* with its surroundings, must of necessity be a very serious matter. It is my province to speak to you of these things; and the problem which I have to solve is—How shall I best fulfil the mission which is involved in my acceptance of this Psychological Chair? Not, as it seems to me, by giving you a long and elaborate course of lectures upon mental science—upon what the metaphysicians term " inner consciousness" and " spiritual essences." The tendency of the age is, unquestionably, to undue amplification. My error, at least, shall not be in this direction. For I have before me the large number of lectures which you have been called upon to attend and digest; the immense demands which have been made upon your time and your energies; the varied character of your pursuits and studies. And I do not think I shall be doing justice to you if I extend this course beyond seven or eight lectures. Therein I shall give you a general outline of insanity, a simple classification, a sketch of the most important forms, and the treatment of disease. For more than this, according to your several tastes or future intentions as to practice, you will consult the recognised text-books.

From this, my intention, you will gather that I regard the measure of my usefulness to you as not lying in the number of my words, but in the subjective force and vigour which I can bring to the portraiture of disease, as also in the spirit in which you receive my utterances. Nor shall we be without objective help and assistance. The Visiting Committee of Colney Hatch Asylum, whose Physician and servant I am, have allowed me, under certain restrictions which I will explain to you at the end of this lecture, to give you an insight into asylum life and practice, and to illustrate my teaching here by the variety of maladies to be met with there. I have pledged myself that you will not abuse this privilege. Of course you will not. You are gentlemen, and students of King's College.

This first lecture will be general in its scope, and as comprehensive as I can make it without touching upon any of the special forms of insanity.

1.—*As to the Prevalence of Insanity.*

Now, by the last Official Report of the Commissioners in Lunacy, it would appear that the number of lunatics, idiots, and persons of unsound mind in England and Wales was close upon 57,000; the ratio per 1,000 of the population being 2½. Ten years ago the ratio was not quite 2 per 1,000. This is the "nearest available approximation to the truth" upon official registrations and returns. Yet still it is a debatable and disputed question as to whether insanity is or is not on the increase. Drs. Maudsley and Robertson are on the negative side; but I cannot help thinking there is some fallacy in the statistics which lead to such an inference, and I am disposed to look at the matter in an altogether different light. Apart from statistical evidence (which is often very untrustworthy), our inclination to one side or the other will be much coloured by the meaning which we attach to that conventional term "civilization." If it implies all that our optimists say it implies—the practice of all the virtues and a greater capacity for all that is good and noble—then you will be disposed to hold to the opinion that insanity can*not* be on the increase. But there is another side to the picture. To me, as I view "this vast rolling vehicle the world, the end of whose journey is everywhere and nowhere," "civilization" may but express wear and tear, and high pressure. And the product of these is deterioration of nerve-tissue, and general impairment of our material organizations. You yourselves are sufficiently acquainted with all that is going on about you to have learned that civilization is really a term singularly inexact and indefinite, and admitting of great latitude of interpretation. It involves an improvement, no doubt, of the social wheat; but there is to be considered also its inevitable correlative—a frightful multiplication of the social tares. If our schools and seminaries, and hospitals and churches have multiplied, so also have our casinos and gin-palaces, and betting-rings; the whole area of speculation is a hundredfold enlarged; all the energies of life are multiplied and intensified; and men shriek at each other on the Stock Exchange who used to converse in quieter and less " civilized " times.

2.—*Predisposing Causes of Insanity.*

From what I have observed of insane etiology, I have come to the conclusion that a great many seemingly small and trivial circumstances go towards conditioning a disturbance which ultimately eventuates in disease. Some of these circumstances are unavoidable. For instance—if nature has given you a pair of "bandy legs" you must put up with them, and make the best of them; but by provoking the ridicule of your schoolfellows, they may be a constant source of irritation, and so endanger the integrity of your intellectual tenement. If one has a squint, or a halting gait, or a tendency to blush unduly, he is equally exposed to derision; and it is not everyone who can bear it with philosophy and indifference. Others of these hindrances to smooth sailing are not imposed by nature, but by the thoughtlessness and vanity of your nearest relatives, who, acting with the best possible intentions, or with no intentions at all, bring about the most disastrous results. If I call my son Shadrach, and my daughter Sophonisba, I am doing them an injustice to which they can have no claim at my hands. The patronymics of many of us are sufficiently hateful and hurtful, without further invitation of the Church's aid, to produce nominal disfigurement of individual men. Many a boy at a public school has been ruined by the bantering and bullying to which his name has exposed him. The neurotic diathesis (of which you will hear so much before you have done with insanity) is evoked and developed by the petty teasings of tailless tyrants; but the tyrants were stimulated into action by the thoughtlessness of loving parents and guardians.*

You may call these things trifles, but indeed they are not so; and if you have brothers and sisters marrying, or you intend some day yourselves to marry, a wise reflection upon the possible results of

---

* "What's in a name?" A great deal more than we think of. I knew a youth who was laughed out of life at a public school because his name was Habakkuk. I know a lad at this present time who is justly apprehensive of trouble with his schoolfellows because his initials (J. A. W.) represent JAW. The transposition of the two first letters would have saved him from the attachment of an unsightly symbol, and from annoyances which may affect a sensitive nature for all time. I am happy to observe that the lamented Lord Lytton, in his posthumous novel, "Kenelm Chillingly," makes allusion to this subject, and dwells in an amusing dialogue upon the evil of baptismal names which are "cacophanous or provocative of ridicule." "On the altar of my name," says Sir Peter Chillingly, "I have been sacrificed;" "it has been a dead weight upon my intellectual energies."

eccentric nomenclature may preserve you and your children from much unnecessary sorrow.

It is known to you that the great secret of successful horticulture lies in ascertaining the treatment required by different plants—their temperature, their atmospheric surrounding as regards moisture and light, and the nature of the soil which they can best utilize and appropriate to their individual needs. Now, just the same care and judgment are required in that social garden which we call the world. The natures of the young must be studied—their parental antecedents (where practicable), their proclivities, their temperaments, their habits, their talents, their aptitudes. Without this study there can be no educational success that is not empirical. The present Bishop of Exeter, and the present Master of University College, Oxford, are noble instances of what can be achieved by force of character and discernment in the culture and training of individual minds. I say it as a layman, and as an alienist physician, that no one can over-estimate the obligations which the age is under to those who have so nobly sustained the previous reputations of Rugby and Marlborough. Such men raise up a barrier against the *neuroses* by co-ordinating and blending into harmonious working the "morality of clean blood," and the morality of the Christian life.

And if this study and this discernment are so essential with natures which, however different, are supposed to be up to a healthy standard, how much more are they required where there is any tendency to run into the morbid and abnormal? The potentiality of example is great; and it is our first duty as physicians and philosophers to counsel the removal of young persons from all those surroundings which are favourable to the development of latent mischief, as in the case of a bad ancestral type.

I have written elsewhere, and I here repeat, "A nervous child should be placed in a strong-minded family; that is, with those who have the *will* in complete domination, never allowing themselves to be betrayed into doubt or vacillation. The melancholy should consort with the cheerful; the unduly hilarious with the more sober-minded and sedate; the wandering and vacant should be won to interest by comparatively sensational modes of placing things before them, their perceptive and reflective faculties being alike encouraged; above all, the timid and introverting, having exaggerated religious feelings, should be placed with one of the school which is muscularly Christian and philosophically Socratic. These adjustments of individual temperaments are the basis of true education, both in those who have and in those who have not passed the line of mental integrity; and society owes all her well-being to their observance. Each plant to its own peculiar soil: thus only can we discern its capacity for growth and beauty."

Believe me, these things are worth considering.

To neglect them is to repudiate the basis of a true and lucid psychology; to study them is, or should be, the power to prevent evil.

In some cases, indeed, your knowledge will only be a power to modify or temporarily suspend the inevitable. In a large number of persons the hereditary law is so overpowering and imperious, that there is no alternative but to yield to its behests. "Multitudes of human beings (says Dr. Maudsley) come into the world weighted with a destiny against which they have neither the will nor the power to contend; they are the stepchildren of nature, and groan under the worst of all tyrannies, the tyranny of a bad organization." Against such a state of things you are powerless. And this sense of powerlessness must, in the very nature of things, lessen your estimate of individual importance. The units, it would seem, are nothing; the totality is everything.

"And the individual withers,
And the world is more and more."

Now, where this bad organization involves what Dr. Anstie calls the active or dormant hereditary neurosis, or what we term the insane temperament, the future of its subjects cannot be very bright or cheering. There is about them a want of uniformity; their cranial development is not always satisfactory; the features are irregular, one part of the face being bright and expressive, another part very much the reverse. They are given to facial twitchings, an occasional squint, convulsive movements of the limbs; all the actions are ungainly, and lack that muscular co-ordination which is the life of symmetry. In early life they may have stuttered, or had occasional fits; and it is somewhat singular that they may have been unusually stupid or unusually precocious. By only "thin partitions" are the two states represented by these terms separated. Those who are charged with any form of neurosis are easily tilted off their equilibrium; eager, excitable, impetuous—they are constantly throwing off electric sparks. They jump and dance, rather than walk, through life. The puberty of these creatures is premature; the sexual appetite is strong, and they are given to habits of self-abuse, initiated either by bad example or the innate impulses of an erethistic temperament. Anyhow, the effect is to aggravate their morbid condition. Happily, the power of propagation is not commensurate with the intensity of their lust, and there is a tendency in all faulty organizations to die out, and become extinct.* I

---

* It is equally singular and instructive, as bearing out the asserted league between a high order of intellectuality and the neurotic temperaments, that the fecundity of both should be defective. "Lord Houghton, in a well-turned speech at the centenary in honour of Miss Hope Scott, the sole survivor of the line, mentioned the kind of loneliness in which the names of all the great *littérateurs* stand. They have rarely left descendants. We have no Shakspeare, no Milton, no Bacon, no Newton, no Pope, no Byron. Italy has no Dante, no Petrarch, no Ariosto, no Alfieri. Germany has no Göethe, no Schiller, no Heine. France has no Montaigne, no Descartes, no Voltaire, no Lamartine. There is no descendant known of Luther, Calvin, or John Knox. The

need scarcely tell you that intermarriages with such should in every way be discouraged. It is a dreadful calamity—the repetition of an insane or a neurotic temperament. The young men and women of our day (and I suppose it has been the same in every day) are too much given to marry without inquiry as to the healthy antecedents of those with whom they ally themselves. Mothers naturally enough conceal their daughters' ailments, and a man finds, when it is too late to turn the discovery to advantage, that he has plunged into the arms of hysteria (which is a neurosis), or leagued himself with an indolent or flatulent female addicted to rhubarb and red lavender. But there can be no excuse for you, as physiologists and men of science, getting into this sort of trouble. You would not buy a horse without a warranty, or attempt to breed cattle without starting with a healthy stock. Be cautious and intelligent observers, and your eyes will soon light upon something which will indicate to you safety or danger. I do not ask you to receive as wisdom the satire of Leibnitz, who said—"Marriage is a good thing, but a wise man ought to consider of it all his life." But I do ask you to take advantage, during your pupilage at King's College, of the suggestion of Balzac, who said—

---

fact is remarkable, and not favourable to the theory of an indefinite progress of humanity. The race of the very great does not multiply, while the race of the very little—say any Irish hodman [or English curate], is as the sands of the sea."—*Spectator*, Aug. 12, 1871.

"Every man should have dissected at least one woman before he marries."

If a faulty organization is a desperate, I need scarcely tell you that a sound organization is a splendid, heritage. It is the greatest of natural gifts, for which one cannot be sufficiently thankful to his ancestors. The somatic integrity of some is so great and continuous that they resist everything in the shape of morbific processes. Like the son of Peleus, they have been dipped in some sanitary Styx, and washed with invulnerability.

3.—*The Hereditary Nature of Insanity.*

This question has already been incidentally touched upon in our remarks concerning temperaments and education. Esquirol has remarked that of all diseases insanity is the most hereditary, and that it is more frequently transmitted through the mother than the father. No doubt a check will be put upon this tendency by the strong-minded women who, dissatisfied with their natural position, and the social arrangements of many centuries, are now striving to make themselves men. Anyhow, the more frequent transmission through the maternal channel will more than justify the remarks which I made just now as to a prudent selection from the many candidates for the nuptial bed who will in due course present themselves to you.*

---

* For my own part I could wish to see these (so-called) strong-minded women lay to heart what a great thinker and writer has written

4.—*Prevalence in the Two Sexes—and in Town and Country.*

There has been a great difference of opinion as to whether insanity is more frequent in the male or in the female, and the large aggregation of women in our different asylums has led to a belief that they are more obnoxious to mental alienation than ourselves. But a source of fallacy is obvious; *existing* cases do not represent *occurring* cases. Women do not die and do not recover as we do; hence they accumulate. It is pretty certain that the *occurring* cases in the two sexes are about equal; perhaps an excess slightly obtains in the males. Insanity occurs more

concerning their crazy appetite for unsexing themselves. "Woman (says Nathaniel Hawthorne) is the most admirable handiwork of God, in her true place and character. Her place is at man's side. Her office, that of the sympathizer; the unreserved, unquestioning believer; the recognition, withheld in every other manner, but given, in pity, through woman's heart, lest man should utterly lose faith in himself; the echo of God's own voice, pronouncing 'It is well done!' All the separate action of woman is and ever has been, and always shall be, false, foolish, vain, destructive of her own best and holiest qualities, void of every good effect, and productive of intolerable mischief. Man is a wretch without woman; but woman is a monster without man as her acknowledged principal! As true as I had once a mother whom I loved, were there any possible prospect of woman's taking the social stand which some of them—poor miserable abortive creatures, who only dream of such things because they have misused woman's peculiar happiness, or because nature made them really neither man nor woman!—if there were a chance of their attaining the end which these petticoated monstrosities have in view, I would call upon my own sex to use its physical force, that unmistakable evidence of sovereignty, to scourge them back within their proper bounds!"

frequently between the ages of 30 and 40 than any other decade. It is more frequent in the summer than in the winter months, and among the agricultural than the town populations. Regarded superficially the latter circumstance is somewhat puzzling, and in contradiction to what one would naturally expect. The vices and the wear and tear of great cities, with all the attendant evils of dense gregariousness, would seem to invite disease in a larger ratio than in the country. But I take it, as a rule, an agricultural is worse fed than a town population. The cold and comfortless apathy, due to imperfect nutrition, of many of our farm labourers and their families is probably owing to this fact. The glorious hills, and the sunny valleys, and the invigorating air are not advantages sufficient to compensate for the loss of that which supplies nerve and muscle, animal heat, and vital energy. Children half-clothed are turned into fields to frighten crows from sunrise to sundown, a hunch of bread being their only sustenance, and they never get really warm from November to June. Animal food is unknown to them as an article of diet, though fat hogs and fatter yeomen are about them everywhere. Starved and stunted and congealed, they cannot learn; but they live to marry and be given in marriage, and repeat themselves in even a less promising form—if that were possible. No doubt the form of insanity to which the agricultural labourer is liable is of a less acute kind (dementia and imbecility) than that of the busy artisan. It is worthy of note that the agricultural counties in which the wages of farm labourers are lowest—and a considerable part of those wages are represented by an allowance of alcoholic beverages (commonly cider)—have a higher ratio of insanity than any other.

5.—*The Exciting Causes of Insanity.*

The causes—the exciting causes—of insanity are, I need scarcely tell you, very varied, and comprised under two heads—physical and moral—of which the latter are by far the most productive. But it is not always easy to define with anything like accuracy the factorship of mental disease; and it is only right I should tell you that my experience of asylum statistics is that they are utterly unreliable. Let me illustrate this unreliability, and point out the reason of the same.

An insane person, who may have been ill six months, is taken to the workhouse. He is kept there for a few days, when, being found unmanageable, he is transferred to the county or borough asylum, on the certificate of the medical officer whom the attesting magistrate may happen to call in. In this certificate a statement is required as to the duration and the cause of disease; and without any inquiries being made on these important matters, the *duration* is commonly dated from the day of the patient's admission into the workhouse, while the *cause* is written down as " unknown."

The mistake is obvious to the experienced alienist, and our accuracy is at once confirmed on the patient's friends visiting him at the asylum.

I have over and over again admitted patients far advanced in general paralysis, the duration of whose malady has been certified as seven days. We have no power to alter the record, and it goes, with many other lies, to make up our statistics, which are really nothing more or less than formulated falsehoods.

In another way, though to a less extent, and in a less culpable (because partly unavoidable) manner, the element of unreliability is introduced in connection with causation. As thus:—

A man holding a good situation, upon which his family is dependent, from some cause or other loses it. No longer a bread-winner, he desponds— becomes the subject of melancholia, and is certified as insane from a *moral* cause : loss of employment. But the loss of employment had already involved a diminished supply of food before the insanity manifested itself, and thus physical privation may have led to his despondency, and been the real factor of his disease. Probably both causes contributed to his unhappy condition, but the exacting requirements of tabulation render imperative our adoption of the physical or moral columns in our statistical return.

Again, a man loses his wife or child. In a month he is insane, and his insanity is assigned to a *moral* cause. But it comes out that the loss led him to drink inordinately; the *physical* element is overlooked, and we write down *moral*. Probably, as in the previous case, both causes had their share in bringing about the mental derangement which has now resulted in loss of liberty and reason. So that the etiology of insanity is beset with difficulties and complications, which limit the exactness of our knowledge, and demand the calmest judgment of the observer.

It is obvious that anxiety and losses, and trouble of every kind, must play a very conspicuous part in the factorship of insanity. Undue pressure put upon the ideational centres in the shape of study is also one of the causal phenomena (it really may be considered partly physical and partly moral), of which we must not lose sight. It is said that the competitive examinations now everywhere established in the public service are telling disastrously upon some of the finer-strung natures. It might be found on investigation that they are of the dormant, if not active, neurotic temperament.

Much evil has been thoughtlessly effected by *fright*. Impress, I beseech you, upon all young persons in whom you are interested the folly and wickedness, even in play, of terrifying their schoolfellows and companions. I am sorry to think that some even of our teachers and preachers need a lesson and a warning upon this subject. Children have been stricken into dementia by the sudden jump from behind a door of a concealed playmate, or startled into epilepsy by an unexpected scream, or thrust into the outer darkness of confirmed melancholia by the "rockets and blue-lights" of a fiery and fanatical preacher. The transition to *religion* as another fertile cause of insanity is not unnatural. There are some I know (and they belong to a theological school which I need not particularize) who affirm that it is impossible for religion to produce mental aberration. Of a truth, I know not why that which contains the largest controversial element of things known to men, and which has produced more bitterness, and cruelty, and bloodshed than anything else in the world, should not derange the world. The fact that it can do and has done these things, and yet, pointing with the eye of faith to the untried and unseen, give to millions unmeasured consolation, is alone evidence of its extraordinary power both for good and for evil.

I should be sorry for you to misunderstand anything which I say upon this very difficult and delicate subject. I should wish you to regard it in a calm and philosophical and unprejudiced spirit; and you will then be led to acknowledge that some minds are so constituted, having such inherited proclivities or acquired tendencies, that, put religion before them how you may, they are certain to make shipwreck of it. The magnitude of its teaching is too much for them. There are others who are repelled by a creed which bristles too formidably with shafts and arrows, but are to be won by gentleness and conciliation. It is the doctrine of verbal inspiration of Scripture, and election, and the personality of the devil, and endless hell and damnation, which are so fatal to the young and the sensitive and the uneducated, of whom I see so many. I could name, if I chose, more than one Nonconformist preacher known for their power to "stain the imaginations of young children," as Mr. Lecky expresses it, "by ghastly pictures of future misery," to whom I am indebted for instructive cases of religious mania. These "foolish and abominable denunciations" (as Dr. Conolly called them) achieve incalculable mischief, and consign many nervous and impressionable subjects to a misery as hopeless even in this life as has been charitably predicted for them in the next.

We turn from the moral to *the physical causes of insanity*.

Without doubt the most frequent of these is *intemperance*. Considering the unreliability of statistics to which I have before alluded, it is not easy to measure with perfect accuracy the extent of this evil as a causal phenomenon. Every additional year of experience confirms me in my belief that it is filling our madhouses with its subjects. I cannot tell you by it how many homes are broken up—how many hearts are broken down. It is a gigantic evil parturient of gigantic misery, committing its terrible havoc not only upon the first, but upon "the third and fourth generation of them that hate Me."

Yet it is to be noticed that even here an element of great uncertainty is introduced. A renowned French psychologist, M. Moreau, says: "Drunkenness is regarded as one of the most frequent causes of insanity. But it is equally certain that drunkenness, or rather *the taste for drink*, is as often, and even more frequently, a first symptom (the effect, therefore, and not the cause) of disease." And this taste, he affirms, has been hereditarily transmitted from the parents to the offspring, just as the same features, and gait, and colour of hair, and complexion. "I receive patients daily at the Bicêtre," the same author wrote, "in whom I can trace back the origin of their malady to nothing else but the habitual intoxication of their parents." These words actually express my own experience at Colney Hatch Asylum. Esquirol long since gave utterance also to something like the same truth when he wrote, "If the abuse of alcoholic liquors is an effect of mental depravity, of educational vices, and the force of bad example, men sometimes give way to it by reason of a morbid impulse which they have not the power of resisting."

Another French psychologist (Morel) also observes: "It is not necessary to create a monomania of which the chief characteristic is an irresistible tendency to fermented liquors. That tendency is most frequently only the *symptom* of a principal disease, especially when it is suddenly developed in persons who previously had given no evidence of such a propensity."

Dr. Anstie, who has made alcoholism a special study, is clearly of opinion that of all depressing agencies it has "the most decided power to impress the nervous centres of a progenitor with a neurotic type, which will necessarily be transmitted, under varied forms and with increasing fatality, to his descendants."

A large-hearted essayist and divine of our own day (Canon Kingsley) has also written, "I am one of those who cannot on scientific grounds consider drunkenness as a cause of evil, but as an effect. Of course it is a cause—a cause of endless crime and misery; but I am convinced that to cure you must inquire, not what it causes, but what causes it."

You see, then, that this subject, in its etiological bearing, is invested with very much uncertainty. The immediate effects of drink are sufficiently obvious, but its ulterior effects are intricate and far-reaching, while the ancestral antecedents of the intemperate may create for them many excuses and entitle them to much sympathy. This subject presents a wide and open field for research and investigation, and I commend it specially to your attention.

Another frightful cause of insanity is *masturbation*, or self-abuse. All alienist physicians bear evidence to the prevalence and power of this pernicious habit.

No vice can be more easily initiated ; none can be eradicated with greater difficulty. "Impurity (it has been well said) can outlive and kill a thousand virtues; it can corrupt the most generous heart, it can madden the soberest intellect, it can debase the loftiest imagination."

It is very remarkable, but it is very true, and therefore I invite your special notice of the fact, that the indulgence of the sexual passion through unsexual means is very frequently associated, in both sexes, with certain neurotic temperaments given to the display of precocious piety and the manifestation of religious ecstacy or gloom.

"I could not say," observes Morel, "how frequently I have seen this pernicious habit existing in youths educated with the most pious sentiments, generally, however, endowed with a timid and retiring disposition." Speaking of this *neuropathia psychica sexualis* in women, M. Guislain says that it finds its constant cure in " marriage and assafœtida."

This subject is too delicate for me to enlarge upon to the mixed audience at an introductory lecture; but you will not lose sight of it, and turn to a profitable account this allusion to the same.

Amongst the other physical causes of insanity may be mentioned injuries to head, sunstroke, epilepsy, childbearing and its sequences (such as prolonged lactation), fevers, imperfect nutrition, and even excessive nutrition—in other words, starving and stuffing. I have often thought that half the world is overfed and the other half underfed. If the distribution of forces could be a little more equalized, there would be less disease and suffering both for rich and poor. The food which I see some persons put away daily is of incredible amount. Heavy breakfasts, hot luncheons with beer and sherry, stupendous dinners, muffins with tea, and just "a snack of something" with a "nightcap" before going to bed! And then—the other side of the picture—how terrible are the sufferings of some from want of the commonest food!

You will now be interested in knowing what are the *chances of recovery and relapse from a first attack* in those who become insane. There is no doubt that the modern treatment of insanity is much more successful than the old system of depletion and purgation. Yet even now the true state of things is sufficiently discouraging.

Dr. Thurnam, who is great in the statistics of mental disease, says that "of ten persons attacked by insanity, five recover, and five die sooner or later during the attack. Of the five who recover, not more than two remain well during the rest of their lives; the other three sustain subsequent attacks, during which at least two of them die." This, of a truth, is a sad state of things, and indicates the immense importance of keeping your upper-storey well swept and garnished—swept from the cobwebs of indolent and degrading obfuscations, garnished by the well-appointed aids of discretion, and temperance, and virtue.

You need not be told that, other things being equal, the recoveries are in the ratio of youth and recency of attack. "The mortality," Dr. Hood says in his statistics of Bethlem Hospital, "as a rule increases with age, but under 20 it is frequently found higher than in the decenniad following, and between 35 and 45 it is much higher than in the years immediately preceding and following."

6.—*Importance of Early Treatment.*

It is of immense importance in the treatment of insanity, as in that of all other diseases, that you should meet the enemy at the very onset; and, other things being equal, the ratio of cures will be in the ratio of the vigour and promptness of your attack. There is a difficulty, however, about the early treatment of mental maladies which requires explanation, and with which you should be made fully acquainted. There is an insidiousness about the approach of many forms of alienation which, even detecting ourselves, we are unable, for various reasons, to demonstrate successfully to others. You can pounce upon a pleurisy and pneumonia, and say, "An open enemy (open by auscultation and percussion) hath done this." My friend and colleague, Professor Johnson (of whose merits and excellence I need not speak in this College) has taught you how to recognise these foes, and how to grapple with them. But turning to the less certain field of cerebral pathology, you will find that it is only in the sudden and acute forms of maniacal delirium that you have a like opportunity of confronting the foe and disarming him of his destructive weapons.

Besides, you may, without offence, tell a man that his wife or child has a pleurisy. He recognises your discernment, and pays a well-merited tribute to your diagnostic skill. But you must be cautious how you tell a man that any of his family are mad. You could not frighten him more, or make him more indignant, if you said they were dishonest. It is almost to filch from him his good name, and stain him with a dye which is indelible. Insanity is a very serious issue. It involves in most cases the loss of personal liberty; it sets in motion the wheels of a costly and elaborate machinery. Doctors, and Magistrates, and Commissioners, and Lords Justices of Appeal, and even the Lord Chancellor himself, come treading upon the scene. It will behove you to be very cautious how you move in the presence of these dignitaries. In stating that a man is mad, you must prove it. You must put it upon paper. You must give all your reasons. A slip of the pen—an inaccuracy as to your own qualifications, or as to the residence of your patient—after you have gone through various processes, will render your certificate invalid; and all your work will have to be done over again. To take away a man's liberty upon the plea of insanity, without complying with all the legal requirements for such a serious step, may be the cause of your being dragged through all the courts in the kingdom. It may involve you in penalties, and loss of character and practice. Even though you are not what are called "mad doctors" (and they are the bugbears of society—especially of the legal profession), yet you will have to do mad work sometimes. I want to tell you of its formalities, and teach you how to do it well.

To return, then, to the question of early treatment, from which this has been no useless digression, and for which, therefore, no apology is needed—let me say that it *is* a great fact, the importance of which cannot be overestimated. But I will give you an illustration not only of the difficulty of being able to initiate early treatment, but of being able to initiate any treatment at all until it is too late. And you will bear in mind that the illustration is a typical one—typical of hundreds and thousands of cases occurring amongst us yearly. The same case will be of twofold value to you, as showing at the same time the inaccuracy of the medical certificates upon which patients are admitted into asylums, and upon which our statistical tables are subsequently based.

W. L., aged 29, married, a costermonger, was admitted into an asylum on December 23. Duration of existing attack *stated to be two weeks.* Supposed cause—cold, and *through a fit.* The facts observed by the medical man, and made the subject of his certificate, are thus put:—" Cannot answer questions rationally, believes dogs are under his bed; talks nonsense." It is added that the case is quite recent, and *not complicated with any form of paralysis.* Observe that the patient has been in the workhouse *two weeks*, and, being unmanageable, he was, at the end of that period, sent to the Asylum, the duration of his disease being dated from the first day of his workhouse experience. Immediately after W. L.'s admission, I diagnosed the case as one of general paralysis of not less than six months' duration, and expressed a belief that he had probably had one of the epileptiform seizures so frequent in this disease; that the insanity was not caused " *through* a fit," but that a fit was one of its results, showing the fatal stage to which the malady had advanced. I had little doubt, also, that the man was of intemperate habits. My diagnosis was based upon the existence of the following symptoms:—The patient appeared dazed and confused, with difficulty only apprehending the nature of anything said to him; his gait was somewhat unsteady, from a want of co-ordinating motor power; he had a blank expressionless face; his articulation was "thick" and indistinct; there was unequal dilatation of his pupils; there *had been* a fit.

Now, remember, the case was admitted into the asylum on December 23. Five days later his wife visited him. From her I extract with difficulty the following facts:—" W. L. is a good husband; never keeps me short of money, and is not a drunkard. He is a fruit-hawker, and has always enjoyed good health until *three weeks ago*, when he had a fit." On pressure, however, she admitted that, though not a drunkard, he was in the habit of coming home most nights muddled and confused; that for *the last six months* he had not been himself; he had spoken of the sums of money he had made each day by the sale of his fruit—sometimes as much as £5—when she knew he could not possibly have made more than 5s. His memory had become defective; he had seemed indifferent to what was going on at home, and had talked largely about his prospects. Gradually this state of things became more marked, until the occurrence of the convulsion. Now observe the inaccuracies which have been imported and tabulated here. The *cause* of the disease is registered as a *fit;* the fit was a symptom, a complication, and not the cause, which was clearly intemperance, of that quiet but continuous and systematic kind which amounts to perpetual alcoholism and befoozlement. Again, the disease was manifestly of six months', and not of two weeks' duration.

So far for the illustration of inaccuracy. And now with regard to the difficulty of early treatment.

Supposing I had seen this man four or five months earlier; it is probable that I should have detected the first symptom of general paralysis, and recommended *an altered mode of life*, which in itself would have been treatment. But how is such a man to alter his life? And where is he to find that quiet and repose which, when initiated, might have arrested the incipient disease? To have spoken openly of insanity would have been to arouse the indignation of his friends; to have advised his giving up his occupation would have been to counsel that which could not have been carried out; to have advised his giving up drink would have been to assume the existence of a vice which he would have denied;—in fact, meet the man and his malady how you may, it is clear that you must here find yourself in a minority of one.

The same difficulty confronts you with equal force in the middle and upper circles of society. We, with our experienced professional eyes, can see the danger coming, when it is even but a little cloud, no bigger than a man's hand, and give the note of warning. But friends cannot and will not see it. How should they? It is not to be wondered at, knowing what we do of human nature. And so you get no credit—the rather discredit—for your advice; for, though it involves the immediate surrender of the exciting cause of the disease, it is at the same time a surrender of the means of livelihood and pleasure. "You take my life when you do take the means whereby I live." Thus, you see, early treatment in cases of this kind is absolutely impossible, because you cannot make manifest to the patient himself and to his friends that there is any occasion for treatment at all, much less for treatment of the kind proposed—demanding self-sacrifice, and freedom from the busy turmoil which has become second nature. When the disease, however, which you have correctly but uselessly diagnosed, culminates in a fit, or in some overt act, or in utterly uncontrollable excitement and extravagance, the friends are alarmed; they retrace their steps, and recall the things which you have previously spoken of as evidences of insanity; at last they put two and two together, and find that it makes four! But the time for all active treatment is now gone by; you may palliate and assuage, but you cannot cure. The disease stands before you, as it were, triumphantly and defiantly, and seems to say, "I came, I saw, I conquered!"

I do not know that I can better conclude this introductory lecture than by assuring you that the insane members of the community are, as a class, the best cared for and best protected in the country. In spite of what you may sometimes hear to the contrary; in spite of the occasional cases of ill-treatment (generally greatly exaggerated for sensational purposes by the press) you may accept this as a verity. For half a century and more we have been moving in one direction, to humanize everything that has relation to those who from disease are no longer responsible agents. It is wise and right that it should be so. The gathering together of the loose and scattered madness of the country has been a great achievement. Unfortunately there is now a growing belief that this has been overdone, and that it is better to treat persons at their own homes, where, amongst friends, there can be no exercise of proper discipline, but, on the contrary, a most injurious amount of feeble and indiscreet kindness! But something is due—a great deal is due—to the sane members of the community, and we have no more right to allow them to be afflicted with the obtrusive presence of insanity when once recognised, than we have to expose them to the influence of a contagious disease.

In my next lecture I shall make some remarks on the physiology of the nervous system; on the pathological changes observed after death in those who die insane; propound to you a simple classification; and proceed with the consideration of some of the special forms of insanity.

LECTURE II.

It cannot be necessary for me to say much to you, I am sure, about the anatomy and physiology of the nervous system, for you are fresh from the class of my distinguished colleague, Professor Rutherford. You have learned from him the general structure of nervous tissue, its division into grey and white matter, vesicular and tubular neurine. He has told you of afferent and efferent nerves; of nerves of motion and nerves of sensation; of the telegraphic system by which the behests of the will are initiated and executed; of the important fact that in the convolutions of the brain, consisting of grey or cineritious matter, lies the intellectual power by which man is distinguished from other animals; that the optic thalami and corpora striata—also groupings of grey matter—are the central points, "subservient to the conversion of sensational impressions and volitions into combined movements adapted to the preservation and welfare of the individual, without the intervention of judgment or the proper functions of mind."

I shall merely supplement this teaching by telling you that through a physiological channel only can you approach with any chance of successful apprehension the science of psychology. Discarding all ideas of "inner consciousness," of a "spiritual essence," and the common metaphysical conception of mind, you must accept at once, in its broadest and fullest, and not in its narrow and conventional sense, the materialistic view of this question. The brain is the organ of the mind, and we have no knowledge of the mind but through the cerebral convolutions.

You may take it for granted that no thought, however feeble, can be originated—no idea, however simple, can germinate—which does not involve an expenditure of somatic force. Every manifestation implies and represents the "change or destruction of nervous element." To be mad is to have this central neurine battery at fault. Its faultiness is the secret and foundation of insane pathology.

Dr. Bucknill puts it well and thus: "The brain, like every other organ of the body, for the perfect performance of its functions requires the perfect condition of its organization, and its freedom from all pathological states whatever. Consequently, the existence of any pathological state in the organ of the mind will interrupt the functions of that organ, and produce a greater or less amount of disease of mind—that is, of insanity."

You see, then, how important it is that you should

be "well-thatched," and have your "intellectual tenements in good repair." You see how essential it is that we should not expose the supreme centres of life to any of those influences which are so fertile in the causation of disease. You cannot poison the blood with alcohol, or syphilis, or carbonic acid gas, or impure and mephitic exhalations, without damaging those delicate nerve-cells which, disarranged so easily, are only rearranged by slow and measured processes. You cannot exhaust nervous power, you cannot eliminate all your "pith and availability" by undue study or immoderate sexual indulgence, or any inordinate sensuality, without inviting pathological changes which, once initiated, may permanently impair that complexity of functions whose harmonious correlation and co-ordination may be regarded as the perfection of mental integrity.

The morbid changes found to exist in the brains of those who die insane are very varied and uncertain. In some cases there is evidence of extensive lesion; in others there is little or no appreciable change. You will not draw from this fact the conclusion that there *is* no change of minute structure, but rather coincide with Dr. Maudsley in thinking that the subtlety of nature may exceed the subtlety of human investigation. The same physician says that "the broad result established by pathological observation undoubtedly is that the morbid changes most constantly met with after insanity are such as affect the surface of the brain and the membranes immediately covering it. Of these changes there is no need of discussion to prove that those in the layers of the cortical substance are the principal and essential."

There is no doubt that in all cases of acute mania there is great hyperæmia of the entire cerebrum. The cineritious substance is intensified in colour, and frequently softened; the pia mater is injected and ecchymosed in patches; on cutting into the hemispheres we find them studded with oozing puncta vasculosa. Precisely the same lesions are not infrequently observed in acute melancholia. But in some of the forms of chronic insanity there is, as I said before, scarcely any evidence of disease. Dr. Bucknill says, " A large number of brains of the insane we have diligently investigated with a first-rate microscope. The results appear to us to have afforded no distinction between the sane and the insane brain." He has found fatty degeneration to exist in the coats of the small arteries in "inflammatory and softened parts of the brain-substance," but not when the pathological changes peculiar to insanity alone existed. The experiences, however, of Schroeder Van der Kolk are different. After more than thirty years' experience he says, "I do not remember to have performed during the last twenty-five years the dissection of an insane person who did not afford a satisfactory explanation of the phenomena observed during life. On many occasions I was able accurately to foretell what we should find."

Unquestionably you can predict in many cases, notably in general paralysis, exactly what you will discover; but certainly there are many cases of chronic insanity in which, the symptoms being identical, the post-mortem appearances are very different. At one time you will find the brain-substance atrophied and singularly hard; at another you will find it soft and sticky, and hyperæmic. I have been particularly struck with this difference in epileptics. In general paralysis, and in certain forms of chronic mania, there is thickening of the membranes, a milky opacity of the arachnoid, and occasional adhesion of the pia mater to the cortical substance of the hemispheres. Atheromatous degeneration of the vessels at the base of the brain is common. It is clear, I think, from the careful investigations of Drs. Bucknill and Sankey that pathological changes are more marked and uniform in general paralysis than in any other brain disease. To the adhesion of the pia mater before spoken of may be added sub-arachnoid effusion, patulosity of the convolutions, dilatation of the lateral ventricles, with a rough granular appearance of their lining membrane, and general œdema of the cerebro-spinal mass. Dr. Sankey has minutely described a tortuous condition ("kinking and twisting") of the capillaries of the cortical substance of the brain, and an increase of connective tissue, previously noticed by Rokitansky and other observers. There seems to be little doubt that in general paralysis there is degeneration of nerve-element, both in the brain and spinal column.

The two forms of *ramollissement*—grey and white softening—so commonly alluded to, and thought to be so general, are really infrequent, and are equally met with amongst the sane and the insane. Hydatids and tubercular deposits are very rare.

It will be necessary before we proceed to the consideration of the special forms of insanity, to suggest some classification under which you may arrange, with something approaching to simplicity, the different varieties of disease which have engaged the attention of alienistic physicians. And this, indeed, is a very difficult matter. Scarcely a writer upon this subject but has propounded a new nosology; and each novelty seems to be more embarrassing than its predecessor. No classification that I am acquainted with is sufficiently satisfactory to meet all the requirements of completeness and exactitude. Nor is it likely that any one ever will do this. Of one thing, however, I am quite certain; and that is that your nosological arrangements cannot be too simple and concise. It is impossible, therefore, that I can recommend to you a modern and much-vaunted pathological classification, embodying twenty-five varieties, by Dr. Skae, of Edinburgh; still less can I present to you, except for purposes of confusion, a modification of Dr. Skae's nosology by a young Scotch physician, containing seven classes and twenty-nine subdivisions, one of which is named "starvation madness" (*limopositos*), and another "post-connubial madness"! This sort of thing looks very learned on paper, but, to my thinking, it is very preposterous and pedantic; for, as Dr. Sankey has pointed out in his lectures, it exalts varieties into species, and multiplies simple conditions which are alike in progress into complicated conditions, merely because there is a slight difference in their causation. You may learn more about madness by reading *Hamlet* than by puzzling your brains over this laboured and elaborate literature.

Perhaps I cannot give you a better idea of an absurdly minute and intricate classification than by placing one before you which was propounded by Dr. Arnold at the close of the last century:

I.—*Ideal Insanity*.

1. Phrenitic Insanity.
2. Incoherent Insanity.
3. Maniacal Insanity.
4. Sensitive Insanity.

II.—*Notional Insanity*.

5. Delusional Insanity.
6. Whimsical Insanity.
7. Fanciful Insanity.

8. Impulsive Insanity.
9. Scheming Insanity.
10. Vain, or Self-Important Insanity.
11. Hypochondriacal Insanity.
12. Appetitive Insanity.
13. Pathetic Insanity, including

Sixteen varieties: (*a*) amorous, (*b*) jealous, (*c*) avaricious, (*d*) misanthropic, (*e*) arrogant, (*f*) irascible, (*g*) abhorrent, (*h*) suspicious, (*i*) bashful, (*j*) timid, (*k*) sorrowful, (*l*) distressful, (*m*) nostalgic, (*n*) superstitious, (*o*) fanatical, (*p*) desponding. To this legion of varieties I should like to add yet another, of which Dr. Arnold himself must have been the subject, and term it "classifying insanity."

I confess I am old-fashioned enough to prefer to any other the simple classification of the great Pinel into four grand divisions—mania, melancholia, dementia, idiocy. It the more recommends itself because it was adopted by Dr. Conolly in his lectures at Hanwell, all other forms of insanity being regarded by him as "mere varieties, or complications, or results." To these I shall merely add General Paralysis, which is certainly a distinct and very remarkable disease, although its various phases involve maniacal excitement, melancholic depression, and that fatuity which we term dementia.

Melancholia.

I shall begin by giving you a description of Melancholia, because some amount of mental depression is said by many authors to be premonitory of mental exaltation. In other words (according to Dr. Sankey), if you carefully investigate the history of every case of primary mania, you will find that its early stage was characterized by evidence of melancholia. The melancholic symptoms may only be slight, and there is a subsequent "evolution of mania." As far as my observation goes, I have reason to think that there is much truth in this opinion. Here, then, is a description of a typical form of melancholia: A person of previously cheerful temper, either suddenly, from some obvious, or gradually, from no appreciable, cause, manifests a change in his habits and demeanour. He is indifferent to what is going on about him—has a general feeling of lassitude and depression; he shuns his neighbours and family, and takes no pleasure in society which he has heretofore enjoyed. His natural sleep is disturbed, and he awakes in the morning unrefreshed, burdened with the oppressive thought of another day, and with a growing incapacity both for pleasure and for work. His taciturnity is accompanied by emotional disturbance. He bursts into tears, appears to be absorbed in a gloomy reverie, from which he is aroused only to tell you that his mind is going, that there is no remedy, that he is "lost," that he has no hope, that his wife and family are starving, that everybody is against him. He may have a good balance at his banker's, but he will not believe it, and no favourable calculations and demonstrations on the *plus* side will make him do so. His credit is gone, he is absolutely penniless. All the acts, he says, of his previous life should have been different. He has refused chances, neglected opportunities, done deeds which in their terrible influence are not to be cancelled. The future has no hope, the past has no consolation. His prospect and his retrospect are alike dark and clouded. It is useless to attempt to reason with persons in this state. Self-feeling is so intensified and exaggerated that you cannot divest them of its painful and absorbing reality. You may tell the religious melancholic that there is hope and comfort for all, and assure him of the same by Scriptural passages with which he is already familiar, and which were once balm to his wounded spirit; but it will not do. There is hope and comfort for all *except himself*. He only is consigned to that outer darkness which can never be illumined. " Which way I fly is hell; myself am hell."

With this state of things, involving so completely, though not exclusively, the affective life, you may have hallucinations of sight and hearing. Delusions you perceive already exist; and a very common one is that food can be of no service, that life can be equally sustained, or death equally met, without it. Or there may be a suspicion that the food is poisoned; and under these circumstances there is often great difficulty in getting the patient to take it. It may be absolutely refused altogether. This refusal is often a negative attempt at suicide. More alarming than delusions are the hallucinations—notably those of hearing—to which I just now referred. Voices whisper or loudly dictate. They may be struggled against for a while, and successfully resisted, but at length, perhaps, they are overpowering. Homicidal impulses (rarely), suicidal impulses (frequently), destroy the autocracy of the *will*, and some act of violence is the result.

In all cases of melancholia you must be on your guard against suicide. You are never really safe, for the determined suicide is so cunning and crafty that he will often succeed in baffling the most vigilant precaution, and in eluding the most rigid surveillance.

The common physical symptoms associated with the above are, in addition to sleeplessness, a languid pulse, a preternaturally red (though at times an extremely foul and coated) tongue, costiveness, dryness of skin and hair, with that "peculiar odour" so commonly noted in insane persons. In women the uterine functions are often disturbed. Frequently there is pain in the head, epigastric uneasiness—a fluttering or burning sensation. This is specially to be noted in that form of melancholia termed hypochondriacal, where the apprehensions are more commonly limited to the patient's own bodily infirmities, upon which he dilates with minute exaggeration. Nosologists, including the great Cullen (whose masterly description of hypochondriasis is well known), have always drawn a distinct line between the last-named disease and melancholia proper. But I am persuaded that they so frequently run into each other, that it is perfectly and pathologically accurate to speak of hypochondriacal melancholia. Guislain supports this view, and Esquirol remarks, "How numerous are the cases of melancholy which have succeeded hypochondriasis. How many instances of melancholy arise from chronic disease, and especially from lesion of the abdominal viscera. Hence we give to these affections the term of hypochondriacal melancholia."

The expression of anxiety in the countenance of the melancholic, the knitted brows, the motionless eyes, the worn and affrighted look, tell a tale of mental suffering which may well awaken our sympathy.

And to such an extent are intensified all the symptoms which I have above described in what has been termed acute melancholia, that the entire affective life is completely paralyzed and panic-stricken. Dr. Blandford well and thus depicts the malady: "This form of acute melancholia demands as much as any the care of an asylum. It is hardly possible to keep a patient in safety in any ordinary house, or to treat him with any but the large staff of officers which an asylum supplies. He is not in a state of mere depression or mild melancholy, nor in silent stupor, but he is panic-stricken. In violent terror and frenzy he paces the room, dashes at the doors or windows, eager to escape from the doom that awaits him, from the police who are on his track. He will not sit on a chair, or lie still on his bed, but is incessantly running about, exclaiming that he is going to be burnt or tortured, that the room is on fire, the floor undermined, and everything ruined and lost. He is suicidal in an extreme degree, and may try not only to put an end to himself, but also to harm himself in every way he can —to gouge out his eyes, cram things down his throat, swallow nails or bits of glass, or break his legs or arms in the furniture. Though he will not attack others, like a dangerous paralytic, he nevertheless resists with the utmost violence all that is done for him. He will take no food, will wear no clothes, will not be washed, neither will he remain in bed."

This state of things is very alarming, and full of anxiety to everyone about the miserable patient. It is associated with great depression, is commonly fatal, and runs its course with rapidity, death frequently resulting from pneumonia and gangrene of the lungs.

There is a third form of melancholia, of which it behoves me to give you some account. It is termed *melancholia attonita* or *mélancolie avec stupeur*. In these cases the patient is often perfectly helpless and passive—conscious, indeed, of what is going on about him, but having no power to *will* or execute.

He stands in one position, or moves only in one unvarying manner. He is indifferent to the calls of nature; he requires to be fed, dressed, and undressed. His countenance is fixed, and he seems to be in a deep reverie. This state of passivity may alternate with occasional paroxysms of excitement, when desperate attempts are made at self-mutilation or self-destruction. Dr. Bucknill has well painted the differential characteristics of those suffering from this form of melancholia and acute dementia. From the latter they may be distinguished—" First, by the expression of the countenance, which in melancholia is contracted and marked by an intense although immovable expression, and in dementia is relaxed and expressionless. Second, in abstracted melancholy the patient resists being moved, sleeps badly, and often refuses food; in dementia he complies with the wishes of his attendants, has a good appetite, and sleeps well. Third, in abstract melancholy the bodily functions are more seriously affected than in dementia—the body is emaciated, the complexion is sallow, the skin is harsh, and the secretions generally deranged; whereas in dementia the body often retains its plumpness, and the secretions are little altered from a healthy standard. Fourth, after recovery the patient who has been afflicted with abstracted melancholy is found to have retained his consciousness through the whole period of his disease. When recovery takes place from primary dementia, the past is found to have left no traces in the memory."

The prognosis of melancholia, when it does not attain the intensity of the *cum stupore* form, or the wild frenzy of the acute disease which allies itself to mania, may be regarded as favourable; but the two latter forms are highly dangerous, both to reason and to life. Not inclining towards death, they have a tendency to run into that "tomb of human reason"—dementia.

The treatment of these cases when they are of the most aggravated kind is a matter of great difficulty, which will at times tax all your patience and resources. On the first manifestation of melancholic symptoms it is of much importance to get your patient away from home, but under proper observation. Change of air, scene, occupation, are essential. You must endeavour to divert the mind from the things which oppress it; all the associations must be cheerful; light and pleasant reading must be substituted for books of a serious kind. I do not hesitate to tell a patient who has a morbid craving for depressing literature that I cannot allow him the use of his Bible, because he only misapplies its teaching. It is everything to discourage mental introversion and self-scrutiny—to take the sufferer *out* of himself, himself being a deranged and emotional chaos.

Light and nutritious diet, regular habits, walking and riding exercise, bathing—these are essential.

I will enlarge upon the two latter subjects, for they have a great bearing upon a successful issue. A little brisk exercise, which sends the blood swinging through the capillaries, and produces that glowing sense which is so thoroughly enjoyed by a healthy subject, will do more good than three times its amount more slowly conducted Of course there are many to whom this is an impossibility by reason of age, and various infirmities coincident with the melancholic state; but, when it is possible, make this sharp and brisk exercise a *sine quâ non*. To promote the free action of the skin is of the first importance, for it is frequently dry and harsh—nay, it is almost invarably so. This is one of the reasons why bathing is so valuable an auxiliary in our treatment; for it is certain that there is a defective dermal action in the insane which gives rise, I suspect, to that peculiar odour so common in rooms frequented by them. The existence of this odour has been doubted by some; but I have no doubt of its existence myself, both among the upper and lower classes. Indeed, I am almost prepared to endorse the inelegant saying, that you may "smell a madman anywhere." The time for bathing should be regulated very much by the taste and habits of the patient; but where he has neither, I would recommend an occasional warm bath at night when the disposition to restlessness is very marked. Shower-baths and cold sponging generally are to be highly estimated; but their adoption when the circulation is languid, on getting out of bed in the morning, is in my judgment a mistake. The conventional idea as to the value of bathing at this period leads to the adoption of a system which tells unfavourably upon certain constitutions. I have seen men and women take hours to recover their equilibrium after this cooling process, when the blood-current is not coursing by any means at its highest force. Cold baths of all kinds are most acceptable and serviceable after an amount of exercise which has pumped the blood into the capillaries, developed animal heat, and unloosed the pores of the skin. The greater your body temperature when you have a cold bath the better can you bear it, and the greater is the thrilling reaction which follows. This is why the Turkish bath is so valuable an agent. Its importance in the treatment of melancholia cannot be overrated, and I am certain that the duration of that state is much shortened by it. It fulfils all the desired conditions above spoken of. The hot chamber produces abundant elimination; the manipulations of the shampooer rid the skin of an immense quantity of dead epithelium, rendering the muscular system supple and pliant; and the concluding processes of hot and cold water complete a renovation which constantly astonishes the patient himself.

You will find, I think, that attention to these matters of bathing and exercise will more or less rectify any abnormality of secretion, and indeed of excretion likewise. Women are more prone to a costive habit of body than men, and you must try and put them right in this respect. But it is a very difficult matter, for so many of them have acquired, from indolence and the use of drastic purgatives, a confirmed habit of constipation. The functions of the uterus must, obviously, not be neglected; and you know the general principles upon which we assail that capricious organ—the home of hysteria—the nursing-ground of embryotic life.

Sleep, "tired nature's sweet restorer," must be courted by every possible means, for the nights of the melancholic are generally worse than their days, and you find them in the morning unrefreshed and unsatisfied. Often better than any opiate is a glass of sherry on going to bed, with some warm and digestible nutriment—arrowroot or sago. Dr. Conolly used to speak of the good effect of this nocturnal stimulant; and, like most of the things which he said, it was wise and prudent. Failing this, you had better give a dose of the hydrate of chloral, twenty or thirty grains. But you must be careful about this remedy. Some are intolerant of it, and I would advise you not to repeat it if any bad symptoms follow. Formerly I used to give occasional doses of one drachm; but I am persuaded that it is not safe—more, that it is highly dangerous. Heretofore, as you know, opium was the great remedy; but it has been greatly overrated, and it is not to be compared to chloral as a hypnotic.

The former depresses and vitiates the secretions, often producing nausea, headache, and costiveness. Chloral is free from these objections. Indeed, I regard chloral and digitalis (the use of which I shall point out to you by-and-by) as the great weapons of our therapeutic armoury in attacking the diseases which are recognised as insanity.

But what are you to do if (as often happens) your patient will not take what you prescribe for him? He may clench his teeth and refuse to take any drugs. In such case you had better inject a third or half of a grain of one of the salts of morphia by the skin. This is much easier in a patient who resists and is violent than throwing up chloral by the rectum—a practice which some speak of highly, but of which I have had no experience. Digitaline may be also hypodermically injected; but remember this alkaloid is highly dangerous and rapid in its action. I had a case of intermittent mania where as much as one grain was borne easily. Less than this produced greater excitement.

When the type of melancholia is simple and passive, unaccompanied by panic or paroxysmal excitement, you may be able to treat the patient at home, though change of air and scene is always desirable; but when the graver symptoms appear, and food and medicine are resisted, and suicidal tendencies manifest themselves, you must resort to an asylum. There only can you insure that organized vigilance and care which are the patient's best protection, and free yourselves, as private practitioners, from enormous responsibility. Obstinate refusal of food is one of the trying and embarrassing complications of the aggravated form of melancholia. You must resort to artificial feeding. A mixture made of Liebig's extract of meat, eggs, milk, and wine or brandy may be thrown in by the stomach-pump. Sometimes a single feeding will be enough, the patient finding the operation so unpleasant that he will not by continued refusal invite its repetition. At other times there is great persistence of refusal, and violence withal; but a little manœuvring and taking the enemy unawares will almost invariably succeed. There have been various suggestions as to the best mode of artificial feeding. Some use the ordinary stomach-tube (as I do), affixing a funnel to the top, and pouring in the food from a jug; others say it may all be done gradually by a spoon process; others, again, introduce a small flexible tube by the nostrils, through which the food is injected from an india-rubber bottle. *Chacun à son goût.* As long as a man has got a mouth, and it can be opened (and I have never seen one that could not be opened), I shall continue to regard it as the legitimate highway to the stomach. The irritation produced by the nasal tube is often terrible. The stomach-pump, when dexterously introduced, seldom irritates, and it enables you rapidly to accomplish what you desire; the whole thing may be done in a couple of minutes. Sometimes patients get an idea that they cannot swallow, and invite you to feed them artificially. I had a tall, scrofulous, nice-looking youth under treatment for delusional mania, whom we had, with occasional short intervals, to feed artificially for nearly two years. Ultimately he died, as might be expected, from inanition. Where, under great excitement, a patient refuses to take his medicine, the avenue to his stomach by the nostrils is perhaps the most satisfactory.

In all cases of melancholia, from the simplest to the most aggravated, it behoves you, as I said before, to be on your guard against suicide. Be vigilant against surprises before the deed, and not surprised into vigilance afterwards. Knives and sharp instruments must be out of reach. Pegs, hooks, and prominences which invite the suicidal to slip a noose over them must not be available for his purpose. By rivers and ponds he must not walk alone. The roar of the panting locomotive must not be too near him, or he may rush impetuously beneath its iron and remorseless wheels. Occasionally he will try to strangle himself by his neck-handkerchief, or to suffocate himself by stuffing up his mouth and nose, or to break his neck by driving with his head at full speed against a wall. In the latter case your patient must be under the strictest guardianship by day, and at night he must sleep in a padded room; in the former, the safest and most charitable thing you can do is to fasten his hands to a leather strap or girdle attached to his waist. This is a better form of restraint than the watching of two or three attendants, with whom there may be constant struggles, and consequent liability to falls and bruises. Considering the amount of cruel mechanical restraint which was employed at the beginning of the century, and that it is our pride and boast that we have emancipated ourselves from a system which, giving no trouble, involved gross neglect, you will naturally enough be reluctant to employ any means which savour of an exploded system. To show you how little familiar we are with such things at the largest asylum in Europe, I may mention that at Colney Hatch we have never had such a thing as a strait-waistcoat. But there are cases, beyond a doubt, where some form of mechanical restraint is called for as the best protection of the patient; and I never hesitate for a moment to resort to it if my judgment tells me that it is necessary.

In reference to the suicidal acts of the insane (for you must not assume, as some do, that a man is necessarily insane because he attempts suicide), it may be desirable at once to point out to you their twofold character, because the matter may be brought under your notice by cross-examining counsel in criminal trials. This actually occurred to myself in the trial of the Rev. Mr. Watson, in January last, when, pressed by the counsel for the defence on the coincidence of the murder and the suicidal attempt as strong evidence of insanity, I stated that much depended on the *character* of the suicide. As a rule, the suicidal attempts of the insane are intensely cunning and crafty, and "contain no element of clumsiness." This is an undoubted fact, and led me to believe that, apart from the question as to whether Mr. Watson was or was not insane at the time he killed his wife, the attempt upon his own life was that of a man in his right mind—that is, of a man fully responsible for his actions. No insane person contemplating suicide would *deliberately and coolly* have told his servant that he might want medicine in the morning, and that the doctor was to be sent for.

You will not infer from this that *all* the suicidal attempts of the insane are free from "clumsiness." Those which are done under "impulse," like all acts which are executed without thought, are often essentially clumsy. For instance, an insane person, in a sudden frenzy, will throw himself out of a window, with a view of terminating his life. Nothing can be more clumsy. I saw one of my own patients, habitually quiet, suddenly rush under the wheels of a butcher's cart that was driving by furiously. Nothing could be more clumsy as an attempt at self-destruction, because it was impulsive—that is, thoughtless—and done without any idea of the proper adaptation of means to an end. If Mr. Watson, under the same impulse which led him to kill, had immediately rushed upon self-destruction by cutting his own throat, or blowing out his brains or throwing himself over the banisters, it might have been valuable confirmatory evidence (which was much needed) of insanity. But he set his house in order, methodically arranged his affairs, and drew the attention of his servant to the fact that he *might*, at a certain time, require assistance.

It is well for you to bear in mind this important difference between the impulsive and non-impulsive suicidal acts of the insane, as illustrated in one of the most remarkable trials of modern times.

In concluding this lecture, I wish to point out to you that both in that form of derangement which is associated with depression (melancholia), and in that which is characterized by exaltation (mania), there is a liability to relapse which constitutes the most trying and discouraging of difficulties. You will have already learned that, except in fevers, the liabilities to what we term relapse, and a periodical exacerbation of the symptoms, are by no means usual. In all diseases persons may vary in some sense from day to day, at one time feeling better, at another worse, even when they are unmistakably on the highway to recovery. But in these terrible maladies, which fasten upon the supreme centre of life, you will, as you proceed in your study of them, learn to experience the most cruel disappointment. You have conducted your patient safely through (as you imagine) all the stages of his affliction, and may be congratulating yourself upon his satisfactory convalescence, and the prospect of his speedy return to the outer world. You will leave him at night calm, rational, grateful, and sanguine in the prospect of that home where he shall renew his affections, and be solaced once more by his wife and children. In the morning you are summoned to him, to find that he has attempted suicide, and that he is again in a state of extreme depression or maniacal excitement. He may have destroyed his bedding, daubed himself with his own fæces, or (in the language of Scripture) "pissed against the wall." Again he recovers; again he relapses—maniacal symptoms alternating with melancholic, constituting the *folie circulaire* of French writers.

The prospect of ultimate recovery, you need scarcely be told, is in an inverse ratio to the frequency of these recurrences. Consider yourselves fortunate if you can lead your patient through the shoals and quicksands of cerebral disturbance without any renewal of those graver symptoms which may be said to constitute complete relapse. But remember, at the same time, that too speedy a recovery is very often only a so-called recovery—the symptoms being only suspended to break out again with renewed vigour.

LECTURE III.

The varieties of melancholia or depression are not so great as those of mania or exaltation; the latter, therefore, is more difficult of description. Just as it is impossible to give a satisfactory definition of insanity, it is impossible to give a descriptive account of mania which shall meet all the requirements of truthfulness and exactitude. In one case the intellect — the ideational centres — may be chiefly involved; in another the emotional or affective life; in another the motor functions. There is scarcely a case of mania, whether chronic or acute, which (though nearly all cases have much in common) has not about it some essentially distinctive feature.

Mania Transitoria.

We will first direct our attention to a form of transitional derangement which best meets the true definition of the generic word "mania" (μαίνομαι, to rage), and to which writers have given the term *acute delirious mania*. It comes on suddenly, with scarcely any premonitory symptoms as compared with those of ordinary mania, and sometimes, after running a brief course, it will disappear with equal suddenness. It is a not uncommon sequel to fevers and the acute exanthemata, exposure to fatigue or the sun, child-bearing, or a debauch. The following case will illustrate forcibly this form of disease :—

I was sent for one morning to see a young lady who was described to me as excessively violent and unmanageable, and I was requested to visit her immediately. She was a handsome well-made brunette, 19 years of age, and had always enjoyed good health until attacked by scarlet fever, from which she had recently recovered. She was happy in her family relations, and was engaged to be married to a gentleman who was in the house at the time of my visit. There was no insanity in the family. Two days previously this damsel had suddenly, and without any obvious cause, displayed a petulance and irritability towards her father and mother, and absolute rudeness and indifference to her *fiancé*. She was heard to talk in her bed-room that night, long after the family had retired to rest, and in the morning it was pretty obvious, from her appearance, that she had had no sleep. Her countenance was flushed; she was in a state of considerable excitement, and she refused to leave her room. Medical assistance was sent for, and two local practitioners were charged with the responsibility of her treatment. But she would not be treated; she refused to take their medicines or their advice, and she spat in their faces when they went near her. As night approached she became more excited, and she would allow no one to approach her. They had a terrible night with her: she tore up and down the room in her night-dress, smashed everything she could lay her hands on, spat at everybody, made use of the most disgusting language, exposed her person, and threw out her arms as though to clutch imaginary objects. She took a singular dislike to one of the medical gentlemen, and he really became quite frightened at her, and left the house. It was on the morning of the next day that I saw her. I shall never forget the look of utter dismay and bewilderment upon the countenances of everybody as I entered the house. They were baffled in all their attempts to meet the emergencies of the case, and even the medical man was on his beam ends. As I ascended the staircase I heard vehement declamations and shouts, associated with as obscene language as the nastiest mind could desire. The bed-room was strewn with different articles; one of the windows had several panes broken; a glass which was fastened to the wall over the mantel-piece was also broken; the whole place was a Babel of confusion. Wild and flushed, the central figure, this young, mad, and imperious lady, with dishevelled hair, torn night-dress, and exposed bosom, sat up in the middle of the bed. "Who are you?" she screamed, drawing herself up with a menacing aspect. "Leave my room instantly; how dare you come into my bedroom?" I approached her and endeavoured to take her hand; but, spitting at me, she sprang out of bed on the opposite side to that on which I stood, and threatened to burn down the house if I did not leave. Fierce as a lioness at bay she stood there, with dilated nostrils and heaving breast, the incarnation of ungovernable passion. The friends around were watching me anxiously to know what I was about to do, and how I was going to free them from their terrible bondage. "That will do," I said; "let us go down stairs again;"—and the patient, without speaking another word, kept her piercing eyes upon me until I had retreated. When we reached the dining-room all looked very much astonished, and were evidently thinking I was as much baffled as themselves. But I had seen all I wanted to see upstairs; a glance, and the history narrated to me on my way to the house, had told me what the case was, and what was needed. My continued presence in the bed-room could only be a source of increased irritation to the patient; the sooner I left her, therefore, the better, in order to organize my plans and arrangements. Now, how was I to set about assaulting the strong citadel of this acute disease? First, I selected another bed-room, and completely dismantled it of all furniture except the bedstead itself, which had no canopy or hangings. A bath-room was close by, and I turned on the cold water, threw a sheet into it, and sent for all the blankets that could be found. I laid a mackintosh—which was hanging up in the hall—upon the mattress, and over that, after wringing it out, I spread the sheet which had been immersed in the bath. My proposal was to *pack* this young lady. Returning to her bed-room with my medical colleague, one of her brothers, a nurse, and three female servants, we seized her, and carried her forcibly and with great difficulty on to the bed where the wet sheet was spread out for us. After much labour we managed to straighten her limbs and get the sheet thoroughly round her, followed by about ten or twelve blankets; we then placed a pillow under her head, and a wet towel on her forehead. For half an hour I never worked harder in my life. But there she lay at last, powerless and baffled. It was a great triumph, and she knew it; and the sense of defeat helped to tame her and tone her down into comparative calm. Now, in a case of this kind the wet sheet serves a double purpose. It is a powerful depressor and sudorific, and it is at the same time a very legitimate means of restraint. It lowers the abnormal elevation of temperature, it converts a dry and harsh skin into a moist one, and it places your patient in a position to submit to ulterior steps and processes. It relieves everyone—both patient and attendants. It gives you breathing-time, and enables you to look about and organize your future plans.

It should be mentioned that the room of these operations had one window, with shutters, which we nearly closed; for darkness is a material aid in allaying maniacal fury. In about five minutes after our patient had been packed she asked for water, and it was given to her iced; she gulped it down eagerly, but she refused to take anything with it. I was now told that she had touched no food since the commencement of the excitement—that is, for two days. Having great confidence in the power of the wet sheet, I did not think it desirable to press medicine, though I had some tincture of digitalis in my pocket, and one drachm of it, or even two, would have been a suitable administration. In ten minutes our young lioness was asleep, and breathing calmly. The sunshine which came upon that distressed family—the calm which succeeded the storm and the tempest—were alike evidenced in the patient and her friends, and filled me with a satisfaction which you can well understand and appreciate.

As a rule, it is not desirable to keep a person in a wet sheet more than an hour or an hour and a half; but in this case I felt justified in doing so. At the end of two hours I awoke and unpacked our patient. She steamed again as we unwrapped the ponderous coverings, and I then instructed the females about her to carry her into the adjoining bath-room, and there place her in an open bath which I had had prepared at a temperature of 75°.

She was quite passive under it, and after being rubbed dry with rough towels she was carried back to the room last used, where, in a clean night-dress and clean sheets, she lay down quietly, in charge of the nurse and one female servant. It was now about 3 p.m. She refused nourishment, and immediately fell asleep again, not waking until eight o'clock. She then took a glass of pale ale, some milk and beef-tea, with two eggs beaten into it, and seemed as calm as she had ever been in her life. So I now felt safe in leaving the house When I called to see her the next day her father and mother, overwhelmed with gratitude, told me that everything had gone on satisfactorily; her bowels had acted very copiously and very offensively, without medicine; she had repeated the nourishment according to instructions at regular intervals. She was perfectly calm, but there was one thing on her mind which distressed her greatly. She knew all that had taken place during her delirium,—the obscene language she had used, and the indecent exposure of her person. She was impelled to it, she said, by an irresistible impulse; but the shame of seeing me again, a stranger until last night, completely overwhelmed her. Would I accept her gratitude and not subject her to an ordeal at which her modesty revolted? Of course I would, and did. She had no bad symptoms afterwards. In three months she was married. She has borne children, and the puerperal state has been free from all complications;

but I have never seen that lady from that day to this.

Now, this case is highly instructive in many ways. In the first place, it furnishes you with a splendid illustration of that transitory maniacal delirium—the *délire aigu* of French writers. In the second place, it shows you the importance of active and vigorous treatment, and that the mere exhibition of drugs is no necessary part of that treatment. In the third place, it shows you the importance of not measuring the need of asylum care and management by the violence of the first symptoms. It would naturally have suggested itself to you that if there was a case for immediate removal to an asylum, here it was. But such a step would have been a great injustice to the family, and would have reflected but little credit on the family's medical advisers. The suddenness of the attack, with premonitory symptoms of only two days' duration, the antecedent scarlet fever, the violent frenzy of the seizure—these were my guides to a diagnosis the correctness of which was fully justified by the result. You will not, of course, expect that all your cases of acute delirious mania will turn out like this one. This occurred about eight years ago, and I have not seen more than three or four since of equally rapid and successful issue. In most you will meet with more marked and extended premonitory symptoms, among which will be, notably, illusions and hallucinations of sight and hearing. These hallucinations underlie and generate suicidal and homicidal impulses. There will be alternating intervals of violent delirium and sullen calmness; at times obstinate refusal of food, a foul tongue and breath, constipated bowels, a dry rough skin, and an indifference to personal cleanliness. If this state of things continues for seven or eight days, and your patient is very unmanageable, you will be justified in taking the proper steps for certifying him and removing him to an asylum. There he will meet with an organized and systematic care which it is quite impossible to provide under home treatment.

At times these patients are excessively incoherent and noisy, shouting night and day at the very top of their voices for hours together. This circumstance constitutes one of the chief reasons for transfer to an asylum, if the case occurs in an undetached house, or in one which is close to a public road; for you have no right to annoy your neighbours, and nothing is more annoying than continual shouting. Moreover, it attracts the notice of passers-by, who stand and listen, fancy all manner of cruelties are going on inside, and circulate all manner of sinister reports outside. This condition, in which there is great exaltation and derangement of the ideational centres, may be succeeded by a corresponding depression, evidencing great terror and emotional disturbance. And this latter phase indicates an unfavourable prognosis; for the arrest of supply by refusal of food, and the absolute waste of tissue resulting from great excitement, have a tendency to produce rapid exhaustion. Obviously, therefore, you must do all you can to get nourishment down your patient's throat, and you must invite sleep by every possible means. Both these matters are obviously attended with difficulty if there is refusal to swallow, and the teeth are firmly and defiantly clenched. I have already spoken to you of the stomach-pump. Here is the occasion for its use. I have an inclined feeding-chair, to which I can fasten the legs and arms of violent patients; a broad sheet round the body and a good staff of attendants complete the necessary arrangements. In throwing in food you can also throw in your hypnotic—the hydrate of chloral is the best. Sometimes you may resort to the subcutaneous injection of one of the salts of morphia, of which the hydrochlorate is the more soluble. In the early stage of the disease, before there is any tendency to depression, the hypodermic use of the alkaloid of digitalis is serviceable; but it requires great care, for its action is quick and powerful. From the one-sixth to the one-third of a grain is about the quantity for each injection, but I have seen a patient who bore one grain.

The tendency of this acute delirious mania (as I have before stated), when alternating with melancholic symptoms, is towards death by exhaustion, or towards consecutive dementia. You may expect one of these terminations if there is no recovery within ten or twelve months. Under a prolongation beyond this period all the pith and energy of life seem to be eliminated from that unfortunate who has been driven through the fiery crucible of this fierce disease. With such an issue on the cards, you will have every inducement to prompt and vigorous treatment.

With regard to the diagnosis of this disease: When you are summoned to its first outbreak, you are—and I doubt not always will be—much too wideawake to confound it with alcoholism; but this mistake has been made, and drunken people have been sent to an asylum as mad. But you must be careful not to confound it with delirium tremens. The terrified aspect of your patient in the latter state, the cold clamminess of the skin, the white and creamy tongue, the tremor which has given to the disease its name, the character of the hallucinations—black cats under the bed, persons getting into the house, &c.—these will be sufficiently distinguishing characteristics. One caution also may be necessary as regards the delirium of fever and meningitis. Here, apart from the antecedents, you have less action and less disturbance of the motor functions, low muttering, incoherent talk, great intolerance of light, with pain and heat of scalp, and contracted pupils. Rigors, too, have preceded, indeed have been among the various premonitions. The end is here sometimes very rapid, with convulsions, squinting, and complete coma.

F 2

Acute Mania.

We now proceed to the consideration of that common form of disease known as acute mania. Although termed "acute," it does not begin in the rapid manner of maniacal delirium, without any, or but few and short, premonitory symptoms, nor does it ordinarily run so brief a course. In very many cases, however, the initiatory symptoms are not noticed in relation to a disease about to develop itself, but they are retrospectively noticed and referred to after the disease has forced itself into unmistakable prominence. The friends of a patient can then, upon pressure and cross-examination, go back a long way, and recover circumstances and conditions, unheeded at the time, which have now acquired a very marked significance. And so it will happen, and it constantly does happen, that an attack of insanity, at first stated and believed to be of a few days', turns out to be of many weeks' duration.

There is no doubt that the history and narrative of a good typical case of any malady whatsoever is the best mode of displaying in their entirety those various phenomena which are known to present themselves with more or less prominence and exactness. Such an illustration my repertory was enabled to furnish of what is known as "acute maniacal delirium." I have another, equally at your disposal, of the derangement which is now under consideration.

I was asked one day to see a gentleman who, residing at Manchester, and being a stockbroker there, was staying with his brother for a few days in my neighbourhood. This brother had himself called upon me, and, proceeding with him at once to his residence, I gathered *en route* the following history :—

A. B., married, 36 years of age; successful in business, happy in his domestic relations, a free liver, but not actually intemperate. "He has been staying with me (said the brother) at my house for about a week, with his wife, for change of air and relaxation from business. He has lately had a great deal to worry him, and his speculations have been of a larger and more hazardous kind than usual—so much so as to alarm his friends, by whom he has always been regarded as singularly shrewd and cautious. The wife, ten days ago, not thinking him very well, sent for his local medical attendant, and he advised removal from home for a few weeks. Accordingly, he came here to visit us. He certainly is in a very strange, unnatural condition, so restless that he won't remain still even for a moment. He talks rambling incoherent nonsense all day, and last night he was singing so loud in his bedroom, from the time he entered it till six o'clock this morning, that we none of us closed our eyes. During the last two days he has become mischievous: he picks the flowers and shrubs in the garden, and throws them about; he is constantly removing the furniture in the rooms from place to place; he dances about and jumps over the chairs; and at meal-times he bolts his food ravenously and fiercely. He is getting untidy in his person, and yesterday he tied some bits of coloured worsted in his whiskers, a circumstance which gave him great satisfaction. He is also obscene in his language and conduct; and last night, while we were in the drawing-room with his and my wife, and a gentleman who was visiting us, he suddenly exposed his person. I was so angry that I at once struck him and knocked him down, at which he burst out laughing. He is getting worse daily, and it is impossible we can do anything with him." This was the brother's narrative.

On arriving at the house, I saw this gentleman in the garden with his wife, his sister-in-law, and a male servant, who was there for the purpose of repressing his mischievous propensities. His hilarity and his intellectual disturbance were at once manifested by his coming forward and claiming me as an old schoolmate, and calling me a "jolly good fellow." His incoherence and garrulity were extreme. He told me his opinions, his plans, his intentions, about everything and everybody. He meant to leave Manchester and come to London as the only adequate field for a man of his brains and enterprise. He should very soon make a fortune. He was going to the Crystal Palace that afternoon, to Hampton Court to-morrow, and to Brighton the next day. Indeed, he should buy a house at Brighton; a "marine villa" was indispensable. Entering the house, I now extracted from the wife her account of matters.

It was this : About six weeks ago she thought her husband appeared somewhat depressed for a few days, but she took no notice of it, for she thought the worry of an anxious business might sufficiently and satisfactorily explain it. This brief depression was succeeded by an elevation of his natural spirits, which had gone on increasing up to the present time. He became more restless, eager, and impetuous in what he did; took more wine than usual, was irregular in his hours of returning home; his habitually even temper became ruffled and more hasty; he took less notice of his children, and though not unkind or indifferent to *her*, he was less warm in the manifestation of his affections. The home ties seemed to be trivialities, and not worth attending to. All his desire was to be away from home, and he spoke of business as requiring his attention in different parts of England. At night he did not sleep, but paced his room; he spoke of wild projects—enlarging his house, erecting a billiard-room, &c. Some of his friends on the Stock Exchange now became alarmed about him, and communicated their opinion to the wife. They said he had been speculating recklessly, and without the least regard to the precautions which ordinarily regulated his business transactions. They were sure he had lost money lately, and was living beyond his means—spending and giving away indiscriminately. As a matter of kindness they came to report these things to her. She consulted her medical adviser, with the result before mentioned.

And now for the state of things which I found existing. A. B. looked wild and excited, and his eyes were clear and brilliant; he was exceedingly talkative and incoherent, rambling from one subject to another, and he was evidently rife for any fun or mischief. His person was untidy; his necktie was all on one side, his hat and clothes were unbrushed, he had not shaved for several days; he kept spitting as he talked; he would not be still for a moment; his breath was foul, his tongue and his teeth were alike coated. I told him I was a doctor, that his friends thought he was not very well, and had asked me to see him. He laughed at this idea, said he wanted no humbugging doctors, and that he was going to London by the next train.

Now I saw at once that this gentleman was becoming very unmanageable, and he would be likely to get violent if all his wishes were not complied with. He had been ill, remember, for close upon two months, and now he was taxing his friends far beyond their capacities to meet his wants, for he was not to be trusted alone for a single moment. So, pointing out to them the nature of his malady, and the certainty that matters would now rapidly get worse, I obtained their ready consent that he should be placed in a private asylum, where I am in the habit of sending patients who are not to be managed at home. I returned to my residence, filled up in the usual mode one of the blank forms of admission to this private asylum, telegraphed to the resident medical officer to send a carriage and two attendants at four o'clock to the house where I had visited this gentleman, instructed his friends to send for a local practitioner to see him at once and fill up the second certificate on the admission-paper, and so placed all things *en train* for protection and security. At four o'clock precisely he was sent for, and removed under misrepresentation as to his destiny. It is quite lawful, and it is a very venial offence under such circumstances, to tell your patient that you are going to Covent-garden Theatre, or the Bank of England for some money, or to any more inviting place than a lunatic asylum. Now, the course which the disease ran in this case was as follows:—On the very night of his removal he became violent, noisy, and destructive, tearing his bedding and hammering at the door of his chamber, —so much so that it became necessary to give him strong quilted rugs in lieu of sheets and blankets, and place him in a padded room. Subsequently he became dirty in his habit, urinating on the floor, smearing himself with his own fæces. This is a very common as well as a filthy practice, sad to reflect upon as indicating the depth to which the cleanly and refined may be lowered by the devastation of disease. For the " dignity of human nature " is temporarily substituted its nastiness and degradation. After several weeks this gentleman improved, and seemed to be on the highway to complete recovery; but he had a relapse, and became as bad as ever, and this occurred three times before the convalescence pushed itself into a less unstable condition, and resulted in complete restoration to health and liberty at the expiration of seven months.

The promising features about this instructive and typical case were—that there was no hereditary taint of insanity, that the cause was clearly excessive mental strain in business, and that the delusions, though marked, were neither uniform in character nor persistent. The delusions which gave an unfavourable aspect to a case are of a different kind: they are immovable and fixed, relating to the same point and subject—they indicate an undoubted lesion of one or more of the ideational centres. The younger your patient, other things being equal, the better your chance of pulling him through; and you will be guided in your prognosis by the circumstance of the attack being primary or otherwise.

After a delusional persistence of twelve or fifteen months, you may begin to think unpromisingly of the case. The maniacal storm has so impaired the intelligence as to make it pretty certain that it can never resume its sway. Henceforth the intellectual life is negative—fitful and uncertain, perhaps, but altogether negative. I have seen a case recover after seven years, but such cases are rare and exceptional; ordinarily, after two years they run into that condition which embraces such a large class of our asylum inmates—chronic mania, with alternating periods of excitement or depression; or the depression may be the leading feature, and confirmed melancholic dulness the result; or acute mania may lapse without intermediate stages into confirmed consecutive dementia. Death, you will say truly, is far preferable to this sad state of things; and indeed it is.

It is better, I take it, after giving you a description of a good typical case, to point out at once the most desirable treatment. In that which I have just narrated the first thing was to obtain sleep. As a rule, it is very desirable to get the bowels thoroughly cleansed by castor oil, or a black draught, or calomel and colocynth pills. When there is great and abnormal heat of skin, with intense excitement, you may (especially in warm weather) resort to a wet sheet; patients sometimes enjoy it greatly. You may also use a warm bath at bedtime, pouring cold water on the head at the same time. I have almost ceased to give opium at night; digitalis where the pulse is quick and bounding, or under the opposite conditions chloral, are far preferable. I have told you before of the power of this latter drug as a hypnotic, and its freedom from unpleasant sequences. It does not produce, as opium so often does, dry and parched tongue, with headache and constipated bowels, and occasional nausea. If it leaves behind it on the following day (as it sometimes does) a sense of drowsiness, you must not repeat the dose till bed-time again, and even not then unless wakefulnes and restlessness have re-asserted themselves. Certainly, when chloral first came out I had several cases in which, having given large doses (from forty-five to sixty grains), I induced symptoms which greatly alarmed me, and nearly proved fatal. As I said before, when your patient has a quick and bounding pulse, you will find two or three drachms of tincture of digitalis more serviceable than chloral. It is not so certain in its action, and in the general run of cases it requires repetition. But, remember, that some persons are very intolerant of this drug, and are easily nauseated by it. I do not regard the bromide of potassium as a hypnotic in single doses. It is more suited to the excitement of chronic and epileptic mania, and must be persevered with three times daily to produce a real effect. In tartarized antimony—an old remedy once much in vogue—I have no faith, nor in Prussic acid, nor in Indian hemp; but the latter drug, in combination with chloral, is sometimes efficacious. With these remedies at night, you must induce your patients to take some light and nourishing food. A little brandy and sago, or beef-tea with arrowroot and eggs beaten into it—these are much-to-be-desired adjuvants. An empty stomach invites sleeplessness as much as an overcrowded one invites the nightmare. Eschew the two extremes : the happy medium is the thing required. Frequently there is a great disposition to tear the bedding and strip off every article of clothing, tying it up in fantastic knots. Under such conditions you must fasten a strong canvas shirt on to your patient by a lock and strap at the back of the neck. There are objections to this, for I have seen a patient half strangle himself in his efforts to pull the shirt over his head. In cold weather, when there is this determined stripping and destructive propensity, you may often advantageously keep the patient all night in a strong canvas suit which laces up behind. In the summer time it does not so much matter; for which of us is not at times during the summer nights in a state of nudity from choice? Strong rugs must take the place of ordinary clothing, which is sure to be torn up as so much paper. From observations made with the thermometer, there is reason to think that very commonly under maniacal excitement this tendency to denudation arises from a dermal hyperæsthesia, which renders the surface of the body intolerant of clothing. Patients have informed me after their recovery of the satisfaction which they felt and remembered in having got rid of every article which encumbered them and interfered with their complete freedom. But you must lay aside the lessons which are to be learned from such facts. It will be your duty, in conformity with public opinion, which is always so just and temperate, to act in disregard of these experiences. It is not prudent to defy her, for, whether right or wrong, she has a majority at her back, and will beat you. In continuation of the subject of treatment, let me add that the bowels must be kept regular; the supply of food must be abundant and nourishing, for there is great waste of tissue going on during these periods of excitement. It is instructive to notice how often in chronic cases the weight of the body rises and falls with the measure of excitement. The more passive the condition, the greater the obesity. Exercise must be regularly attended to; much superfluous energy may be got rid of by judicious athleticism. Cold bathing—shower-baths in the summer—an occasional pack under exceptional excitement—are health-giving and restorative. The Turkish bath is not adapted to cases of mania as to those of melancholia. Sudorification is sometimes very difficult of attainment, and the hot chamber irritates without opening the pores of the skin. Besides, there is the risk of a patient injuring himself, becoming violent, and getting in contact with the hot surroundings. A vapour bath is much better for mania than a hot-air bath.

These are the means by which we endeavour to combat acute mania, and look expectantly for recovery. It is pleasant beyond all description to hail the dawn of a long occulted reason, to welcome back the first silver streaks of returning day. It is encouraging to see the afflicted resume their interest in the things about them, inquire after friends, occupy themselves rationally, desire to make themselves generally useful, express a wonder as to what has been going on about them, and a suspicion that their fancies were *but* fancies, for the absurdity of which they are unable to account. The best evidence of improvement is when, having had delusions, your patient now admits that they *were* delusions; or, having been beset by hallucinations, he now hears no more voices and sees no more figures by his bedside at night. All the functions of body and mind are now healthfully progressing. At this period the Turkish bath will be of great service, and rapidly expedite the cure.

Simple Mania.

I propose now to speak to you of a certain class of persons to be met with, both in public and private practice, who, without presenting any acute symptoms either of exaltation or depression, may be fitly termed maniacal. We are consulted about them by their friends for strangeness of ideas and conduct. They have delusions, about which they talk pretty freely; and sometimes these delusions are of a kind which may lead them into trouble if some restraint is not put upon their actions. This state of things may have been gradually coming on for a considerable period. Sleep now becomes impaired, appetite fails, regularity of habits is interrupted. Change of air and scene, withdrawal from every exciting cause of disturbance, in the companionship of a judicious friend, with general attention to health, a few Turkish baths, and a few doses of chloral at night, will generally in a few weeks restore these cases. We term these patients, I repeat, maniacal; their intelligential centres are disturbed, their affective disposition being for the most part unimpaired. It is often necessary, especially among the lower classes, to move those who are thus deranged to an asylum. They do not like this; they resent it, threaten legal proceedings, and are disposed to give a good deal of trouble. But they often recover quickly after this imposed retirement of a few weeks' duration. In some cases there is a premonition which amounts almost to a brief stage of dementia. I have frequently admitted patients, commonly young men, who have appeared for a few days to be completely vacant—dazed, as it were, by the light of the "garish day,"—stunned, it may be, by the noise and bustle and everlasting spin of this fast six-mile-cannon age. In a few days they wake up from their temporary torpor; they may then have delusions; wonder why they are detained, and where they are, and manifest great impatience for their discharge. These cases commonly do well, and are by no means of long duration. Their appearance, at first, would not lead you to suppose they would so soon recover.

Not unfrequently there is one fixed idea in the mind, founded upon a false impression. This is what authors have termed "monomania." As a rule, what is designated monomania is not so, strictly and philologically. It is doubtful, indeed, whether there is *ever only one point* upon which the mind is unsound. For instance, a man may tell you he is Jesus Christ; and this is the subject upon which he harps, it being ever uppermost in his thoughts. But on pressure you will generally find there is something else in the background. Be this as it may, however, it is hardly correct to say that the man is only mad upon one point, and sane upon all others. Dr. Maudsley has well alluded to this matter: " In vain do men pretend that the mind of the monomaniac is sound, apart from his delusion; not only is the diseased idea a part of the mind, and the mind, therefore, no more sound than the body is sound when a man has a serious disease of some vital organ, but the exquisitely delicate and complex mechanism of mental action is radically deranged; the morbid idea could not else have been engendered and persist. The mind is not unsound upon one point, but an unsound mind expresses itself in a particular morbid action. Moreover, when the delusion is once produced, there is no power of drawing a sanitary cordon round it, and thus, by putting it in quarantine, as it were, preserving all other mental processes from infection; on the contrary, the morbid centre reacts injuriously on the neighbouring centres, and there is no guarantee that at any moment the most desperate consequences may not ensue."

When patients whose derangement commences in this gradual way do not improve after some months of care and treatment, the prognosis concerning them is unfavourable. Their delusions become more marked; they get more eccentric in their ways and general bearing, and nosologically attach themselves to that large class of chronic lunatics with whom our asylums are so thickly peopled, and who evidence moral as well as intellectual insanity. Less sensible of the requirements of order and decorum and the general proprieties of life, they do strange things, and wonder that the term "strangeness" is used by anyone to designate their proceedings. A real idea of their conduct and character is perhaps best expressed by the word *bizarreries*. Their dress is peculiar: gay and ill-assorted colours usurp the place of that sombreness of garb which previously satisfied them; in the matter of hats and the decorations thereof they are singularly ingenious and amusing. These antics and fantastic arrangements of the external man are but the measure of inner oddities and entanglements which go to make up the objective and subjective madman. Much that these subjects do they can well avoid doing if they make the effort; but, like others, who have only temptations to do wrong, and no particular aspiration to do right, they find it hard to keep the driving-wheel of their moral locomotive on the rail—they get jolted, or rather they jolt themselves, off it; and they rather enjoy the disturbance and embarrassment which the jolting process entails upon others. These anomalous creatures must be kept under moral control; you must not let them see that you regard them in any sense as irresponsible agents. You must of course make allowances for them; but you must give them no encouragement, or they will be sly enough and clever enough to take advantage of it, and give you an infinity of unnecessary trouble.

It is of great importance in the management of this large class of lunatics to discover their individualities of character, their weaknesses, their strength, their proclivities. More than half the secret of success in the superintendentship of an asylum lies in the possession of this faculty, and in the due exercise and application of it. If you attempt to talk to one lunatic as you might to another you will find yourself in difficulties. To all you must be kind; but your kindness in many cases must be blended with a cautiousness and a firmness which will make manifest to the patient that you are not to be imposed upon or trifled with. Others do not need this: they live in an atmosphere of subdued gentleness, being of gentle natures; and you must treat them accordingly. Many of the confirmed chronic lunatics in our asylums are constantly fretting for removal to another, where they hope to better themselves by a greater defiance of authority, and by the exhibition of greater tact towards their superiors than they are conscious of having displayed in their present abode. They want to try their cunning upon a new superintendent. I am very careful in my dealings with these gentlemen. I have had patients brought to Colney Hatch who have been grievously disappointed after a few days' residence to find that they have not bettered themselves—that they have got out of the frying-pan into the fire.

When once insanity—be it mania, or melancholia, or acute dementia—assumes a fairly recurrent type, it is almost invariably hopeless, and I believe those authors are correct who state that speedy recoveries (so termed) are very frequently of a temporary and evanescent character; in other words, a person suffering under a primary attack of acute mania or melancholia is more likely to *remain* well if he is some little time in shaking off the enemy than if he succeeds in doing so (or perhaps it would be more correct to say, if it is thought he has succeeded in doing so) with greater rapidity. I have evidence of the truth of this, which seems to be at variance with the law obtaining in other diseases.

The intervals between maniacal and melancholic attacks may vary in duration from months to years; but when once fairly established the periodicity remains pretty well defined. Those who have the longer healthy intervals resume their places in the outside world after each attack; but I doubt if the eye of an acute and experienced alienist physician would not at all times, if thrown much upon them, detect some abnormality of thought or action which would suggest to him an uneasy and insane temperament. The pathology of this continuous but unevenly sustained disease is very interesting to consider; the symptoms, I take it, being conditioned by a local hyperæmia of varying intensity and duration, the causes of which it yet remains to discover.

To that variety of derangement where melancholia alternates with mania, the French have given the name "*folie circulaire*" or "*à double forme.*" As an illustration of the established periodicity of maniacal excitement, I may mention that I have a patient who regularly every seven weeks becomes talkative, noisy, destructive, and occasionally dangerous. The attack lasts for about a week, and is always ushered in by a foul tongue and constipated bowels. The fellow knows as well as possible what is going to happen (for he is fortified by an experience of eight years), and he asks for opening medicine, and insists upon going into seclusion. For a couple of nights he will chatter incessantly; on the third or fourth day he will bury himself under the bed-clothes and speak to no one, though he may be seen shaking with a suppressed laugh or hysterical cry. At the end of eight days he is himself, and he returns to his occupation on the farm grounds of the Asylum, where his work is equal to that of any paid labourer.

Dr. Sankey thinks that in many cases of secondary insanity the morbid processes which involved the first attack have never totally ceased. Smouldering, but undetected, they have really remained, so that the secondary attack is not a fresh pathological condition, but simply a renewal of the first.

About 40 per cent. of the occurring cases in England and Wales are said to be secondary—that is, other than primary; but my own statistics (confessedly unreliable) at Colney Hatch do not give more than 20 per cent. These cases of recurrent insanity are frequently associated with impulsive acts of great violence, such as window-breaking, destruction of clothes and bedding, aggressive attacks upon others and upon self. They constitute a large portion of our insane population, and invite great care and vigilance.

LECTURE IV.

Moral Insanity (so-called).

I HAVE now to direct your attention to a very important form of insanity which, it has been truly said, "more than any other has puzzled the psychologist, perplexed the advocate, and disconcerted the divine." It does not appear that, as our psychological and pathological researches are extended, we have any clearer ideas than formerly of that derangement to which Dr. Pritchard gave the unfortunate name of *moral insanity*—defining it to be "a morbid perversion of the natural feelings, affections, inclinations, tempers, habits, moral dispositions, and natural impulses, without any remarkable disorder or defect of the intellect, or knowing and reasoning faculties, and particularly without any insane illusion or hallucination."

Under the term *manie sans délire*, Pinel had previously described a madness involving no intellectual disturbance, the emotional or affective nature alone being implicated. Subsequently,

Esquirol, with that love of new nomenclature which is almost a professional disease, introduced the term *monomania*, making it, in defiance of its significant Greek derivative, to embrace two varieties—instinctive and affective. Modern writers have still further multiplied varieties and terms, the result being that when this technical phraseology is introduced by a medical witness into our law courts, modern judges become alarmed, and hint to him the undesirability of "getting into the clouds." Fine feathers, it is thought, make fine birds, and I suppose complex divisions and subdivisions make fine nosologies, and convey to outsiders the idea of great erudition.

In whatever shape, however, we may frame our classification, or in whatever words we may think fit to clothe our differential expressions of disease, it is beyond a doubt, as Esquirol pointed out, that moral alienation is the proper characteristic of mental derangement. This great psychologist declares that, whatever the difficulty about detecting hallucinations or delusions, there is no exception to the rule of perversion of the passions and moral affections. This perversion is the substratum of every deviation from the normal standard of mental integrity. "To insist, therefore, upon the existence of delusion as a criterion of insanity is," Dr. Maudsley writes, "to ignore some of the gravest and most dangerous forms of mental disease."

And yet it may be doubted whether, in all cases

of what is termed moral insanity, there is not mixed up some faint element of delusion. For instance, no class of lunatics are so confident in the soundness of their own condition. Here, then, is something very like a delusion *in limine*. Certainly (as Dr. Blandford has remarked) the absence of the moral sense does not prove or constitute insanity any more than its presence proves sanity. " It is perfectly true," he writes, " that it is absent in many lunatics, all notions of duty, propriety, and decency being destroyed in the general overthrow of the mind; but it is also true that we can find perfectly sane people who, either from early education and habit—the habit of continual vice—and also hereditary transmission, are devoid of moral sense to an equal or greater degree. Probably greater wickedness is daily perpetrated by sane than ever was committed by *in*sane men and women; so that when immorality makes us question a man's state of mind, it must be remembered that insanity, if it exists, is to be demonstrated by other mental symptoms and concomitant facts and circumstances, and not by the acts of wickedness alone." It is not to be wondered at that society is very jealous of the admission of moral insanity as a distinct form of disease, and has regarded its plea as little else than a frequent apology for crime, devised by the cunning of " mad doctors." I confess that I have more than once looked upon the distinctions attempted to be drawn by alienist physicians as too fine and too subtle; and to this circumstance I attribute the present unpopularity of those specialists who are supposed from the nature of their calling to regard everybody who breaks the law, through a mad focus. The plea of insanity raised in the case of Arthur O'Connor in the month of April last is not, as it seems to me, calculated to raise us in public respect and estimation.

Your sensational experience in the perusal of the daily press has already made you acquainted with the fact, that what is termed moral insanity, at times derives great and spasmodic interest from its association with great crimes. It is of importance that when brought in contact with cases of this nature you should set at once about inquiring as to the antecedents, both personal and ancestral, of those whose actions you are called upon to judge. And you will very commonly find that there is an hereditary taint of madness transmitted from one or—fatal combination—both parents. If there is not direct evidence of this, there is at least very much to show the existence of a neurotic temperament, either in the shape of what is termed eccentricity, or hysteria, or epilepsy, or some other form of deviation from that stable condition of nerve-element which cannot be too highly estimated, and can never be too sedulously preserved. There is no reason, indeed, why the insane temperament or (as some have phrased it) *diathesis spasmodica* should not be of idiopathic origin. All the ailments to which we are subject must have a starting point, although their full development as a somatic entity is commonly the result of accumulated and transmitted forces, acquiring increasing volume with increasing years.

The characteristics of this temperament are, for the greater part, vanity, restlessness, capriciousness, impulsive action, with general eccentricity of thought and feeling, and not unfrequently a singularly inharmonious physiognomy. If you will let them, the subjects of this diathesis will absorb much of your time and attention, and think you could not be better employed than in attending to them. The groove in which they run has a borderline on either side, mapping off the land of genius and the land of insanity. And when they get off this groove (as they so often do), the odds are twenty to one that they topple over to the wrong side of what has been called the "thin partition." Having no "capacity to establish an equilibrium between them and external conditions," their ideas of achieving greatness are anything but the measure of their performances, which merge into the realities of disappointing littleness. Obviously the outcome of this temperament is largely conditioned by the social and other surroundings of the individual man; so that to one, from serene and gentle influences, will arise the evolution of positive insanity, while to another, from far different and tumultuous dispositions, will be generated a ceaseless provocative to disease.

I have under my eye a most instructive case of this form of insanity, which will be to us its most fitting illustration.

A. B., a solicitor's managing clerk, aged 56, married, with a large family, has always been of an eager, restless, and excitable temperament. No ascertained hereditary taint. Has now for years kept his family in constant hot water, as well as in bread and meat. The supply, indeed, of the former has, I understand, been the more liberal. Is vain, jealous, suspicious, captious, and easily moved to demonstrative anger. After some of these demonstrations he will decline to speak to members of his family for weeks, during which time he will occupy himself with Utopian schemes for their separation or the complete reorganization of his home arrangements. These schemes he will commit to paper, couching them in elaborate legal phraseology. He is singularly neat and precise in his dress and general habits, as also in his forms of speech. He is much given to a weakness for the other sex, and if he passes a nice-looking woman, he will probably take off his hat, fancy she is in love with him, and do his best to gratify his wife by telling her his opinion. You perceive by such traits as these and others, that he has exaggerated notions of self-importance. He makes notes and preserves written records of occurrences relating to his own condition, and surroundings, and prospects. There is an unmistakable alienation of this man's entire moral nature. This state of things is, of course, incompatible with steady perseverance in business. A change is noted at the office in his habits, in his temper, in his manner of taking instructions from his superiors, and of executing the same. He criticises, and almost dictates, where once he submissively performed without doubt or question. He quarrels with his fellow-clerks, and makes everyone about him so uncomfortable that his employers are necessitated to dispense with his services. Matters at home are not improved by this measure, which deposes the chief bread-winner of the family. His temper is greatly aggravated, and he becomes violent and threatening, and is placed in an asylum. The history of the case up to this period is the history of three years. There is, you will observe, as I have narrated and as I have received it, no evidence of intellectual disturbance, but simply a morbid perversion of thought and feeling, an exaggerated self-estimate and love of notoriety. Beyond this the intelligential faculties do not appear to be implicated. But now for the first time—as, according to my experience, happens sooner or later in all cases of what is termed moral insanity—we have distinct delusions. There is not only the delusion that he is not insane (to which I have before made reference), but there is a fixed belief that his family is in a conspiracy against him, and that his son, who has been taken into the office of his late employers as an act of kindness, has supplanted him by false representations. After a residence of eight or nine months in a London asylum, where he was exceedingly exacting and troublesome, he was transferred to Colney Hatch. On admission it was clear at a glance that he was "saturated with insanity." His physiognomy was unmistakable, and such as objective experience, and not verbal description, will alone impress upon you. It was amusing in the extreme to watch my new friend take stock of his new physician. He had evidently got himself up for the occasion; he expected I was going to trot him out, try his paces, and then by a prompt and decisive measure baffle the machinations (as he termed them) of his friends, and confirm his judgment of his own soundness by immediate dismissal and freedom. But there is no necessity to trot out lunatics of this type; they are unconsciously trotting themselves out from morning to night; their whole life is an exposition of abnormal conduct, revealing itself by look and gesture and language, and countless eccentricities, which go to make up that complex form of insanity which we have now under consideration. This individual has now been under my care about six months, during which time he has written me about two hundred letters, some of them long and elaborate, and couched in legal phraseology, their envelopes bearing the word "Important," or "Official," or "Immediate." At times he sends me a document addressed to the Secretary of State and other persons of official distinction, to whom he makes known his case of unjust and "illegal incarceration" (as he phrases it), and appeals for his discharge. When I see him he seriously asks me as to each letter sent, and expresses surprise that he has received no answer. The silence of their correspondents does not deter patients of this class from writing again. They are persevering to an extent which would be highly laudable in a better cause, and their zeal leads them to send out letters by surreptitious means if they can possibly manage it. You should be told, by the way, that all the letters to and from the insane inmates of an asylum are supposed to pass through the hands of the Medical Superintendent. Your experience will soon teach you the necessity of such a measure.

A few more words respecting this illustrative case, and I have done with it. Our friend (as I told you before) is intensely vain, and places upon himself a very high market value. All the women on the premises are, he thinks, in love with him. He is given (after the manner of the morally insane) to what is termed "smutty" conversation, and to acts which trench at times upon the indecent.

Cases of this kind require great colloquial tact and management, the more so as they are commonly permanent institutions. In other words, they do not often recover when the disease is of any standing. They require a happy mixture of firm but conciliatory treatment. You must let them feel the rein, but you must at the same time moderately and playfully humour them.

Sometimes moral insanity is characterized by a great and shameless depravity, of which the above case yields no indication. Women of good social position and education will manifest an utter disregard of all the decencies of life. Spasmodic intemperance and sensuality will for a time destroy all the proprieties which are ordinarily regarded as having imperious claims. Often allied with some form of neurosis, such as hysteria or epilepsy, this distressing malady will give scandal and notoriety to a neighbourhood. Its subjects will break all the commandments of the Mosaic law, and many others (not written upon tables of stone) which society has set up for her protection. In the sex endowed with a child-bearing organ exacerbation takes place at the menstrual periods, and erotic symptoms are very marked. Impulses of depravity will manifest themselves in exposure of the person, in disgusting language, and in various acts of indecency which need not be particularized. So also impulses of violence and destructiveness will be evidenced by broken windows, torn clothes and bedding, and even self-mutilation. At such times women will introduce foreign bodies into the vagina, swallow pins, eat and drink the excretal residua of previous eatings and drinkings, and disclose endless varieties of vitiated taste and feeling. I had a patient who, for purposes of wanton mischief, secreted a large nail in his rectum, and destroyed with it, in one night, a new padded-room. His satisfaction in the morning was charming to witness; his regret a month later, when he was for a few weeks in a fairly normal state, was touching.

Impulsive Insanity.

But I must direct your attention briefly to a form of impulsive insanity <u>in which there is no intellectual disturbance,</u> but yet some abnormal condition of nerve-element which generates a thorough perversion of the affections and feelings. It is of great importance that you should make a careful study of those cases <u>in which there are no delusions proper,</u> for they frequently involve all kinds of medico-legal differences. Formerly the existence of delusions was regarded as the proper test of insanity. But such a test has now no local habitation; even the most obscure legal minds have discarded it. Every experienced criminal lawyer, as well as every experienced alienist physician, will tell you that there are plenty of mad people who never had any delusions. No doubt, in a large proportion of those who have homicidal or suicidal impulses, such impulses result from hallucinations or delusions. But in others there is simply impairment of volition, from perversion of feelings and desires and appetites. <u>With every inducement to avoid a criminal act, and a complete knowledge of its wickedness, one is yet impelled irresistibly to its achievement.</u> There is

H

no relief for the pent-up destructive energy but in an " irresistible utterance of action." " The act of violence," Dr. Maudsley writes, " whatever form it may take, is but the symptom of a deep morbid perversion of the nature of the individual, of a morbid state which may at any moment be excited into a convulsive activity, either by a powerful impression from without, producing some great moral shock, or by some cause of bodily disturbance —intemperance, sexual exhaustion, masturbation, or menstrual disturbance. There are women, sober and temperate enough at other times, who are afflicted with an uncontrollable propensity for stimulants at the menstrual period; and every large asylum furnishes examples of exacerbation of insanity or epilepsy coincident with that function. In fact, where there is a condition of unstable equilibrium of nerve-element, any cause, internal or external, exciting a certain commotion, will upset its stability, just as happens with the spinal cord under similar circumstances. By his acts, as well as by his speech, does man utter himself. Gesture-language is as natural a mode of expression as speech; and it is in insanity of action that this most dangerous form of affective insanity is expressed—most dangerous, indeed, because so expressed."

In giving evidence as to the existence of impulsive insanity in criminal cases, you will be sorely pressed by cross-examining counsel concerning the probability of a homicidal act being the first symptom of a disordered mind. Cases of this kind are very naturally and very properly regarded with grave suspicion by the judges and the public; and I am disposed to think that this suspicion has of late been greatly heightened by attempts on the part of medical witnesses to advance the theory of irresponsibility upon insufficient evidence of disease. Now, of course it is impossible to say with absolute certainty that an overt act of criminal magnitude may not have been the first external utterance of a pre-existing insanity. But the likelihood of such a circumstance is so highly improbable as to render its negative an approximative certainty. These impulsive acts are common among persons known to be mad, and under confinement as such, but not among those in whom insanity was never previously dreamed of. In Esquirol's famous treatise on mental diseases, the subject of homicidal mania is comprehensively handled; and he gives a large number of illustrative cases, in all of which, as I read them, there was unmistakable evidence of insanity prior to the aggressive deed. In the *American Journal of Insanity* for October, 1857, the details of no fewer than fifty-two homicidal cases are placed on record, in all of which previous insanity was undoubted. Dr. Blandford says, "I think you will find, if you go to the root of the matter, that the act which is supposed to be committed under the influence of insane impulse is rarely, if ever, the first symptom of insanity or brain affliction shown by the alleged lunatic. You may be told by friends that they have never seen any insanity in him; but some people cannot see it in five out of the six patients in an asylum. If you can get sufficient information you will probably discover that he has had former attacks, from which he may or may not have been considered as recovered."* Dr. Sankey says, "I have taken the precaution to read a large collection of reports, published from time to time in the *Annales Médico Psychologiques*, upon the state of mind of persons accused of different acts of violence. I have never yet discovered a case in which an act of violence was committed by a lunatic as his first insane act. There are several cases in which the patient was not considered insane by his own relations, or by inexperienced medical practitioners, but who, on the closer scrutiny of the physician who had studied insanity, was clearly proved to have been so for a long period."† I have given evidence to this effect at the Old Bailey in January last in the case of the Rev. John Selby Watson, when of course the effort made by the defence was to prove that the prisoner had already demonstrated by acts previous to the murder his mental unsoundness. But I did not perceive insanity in the acts alluded to, and therefore I pronounced him to be of sound mind.‡

* "Insanity and its Treatment," pp. 329, 330.
† "Lectures on Mental Diseases," p. 97.
‡ This gentleman has now been incarcerated for fourteen months;

You will observe that in this impulsive or emotional insanity the motiveless character of a homicidal act cannot but furnish evidence of derangement, and *vice versâ*. For instance, if a man kills a wife whom he adores, the act is *à priori* more likely to be an insane one than if he kills a wife whom he hates, and from whom he has received the greatest provocation.

There is no doubt that the <u>unstable condition of nerve element, which lies at the root of epilepsy</u>, furnishes some of the most desperate instances of homicide as of every vicious impulse. I have at this time under treatment a very instructive case of masked epilepsy in a boy only thirteen years of age; and, while we are on this subject of impulsive insanity, I cannot do better than present the same to your notice. I had been looking out for an epileptic fit, to furnish the only explanation of the most ungovernable and motiveless fury possible, when on the 13th day of February it came, and the demoniacal rage which had previously been so disastrous was transmuted into a distinct and characteristic convulsion.

J. C., aged thirteen, having nothing normal in his cranial conformation, was admitted into the Asylum on October 7th, 1871. The statement made by the certifying medical officer was as follows:—
"Found him sitting almost naked over the fire,

and to no one about him has he, during that period, given the slightest evidence of insanity.

frying some potatoes and making a knife and fork red-hot, with which, he said, he was going to eat his dinner and stab his mother. States he has a house of his own, and defies the Queen, bishops, magistrates, or police to turn him out under twenty-one days. The mother states that five months ago he ran a chisel down his throat. He has been twice locked up for maliciously breaking windows. A fortnight ago he first used threatening language, and has gradually become worse. On Friday last he attempted to stab his mother and poison her with paraffin oil. Threatens to stab his brother, and also to burn down the house."

Now, this is a nice promising little episode in a life which has not yet run over fourteen years; but you will hear presently of an unpromising history and background which will explain all and invite your sympathy.

Observe, under the mask of epilepsy we have pyromaniacal impulses, matricidal impulses, fratricidal impulses, together with general depravity and ferociousness. For the first few days after admission this boy was excited and savage at being removed from home. Subsequently he toned down into perfect quietness and propriety of conduct, until the end of December, when he suddenly broke out into the most ungovernable passion, attacking everyone within reach, and using the foulest and most blasphemous language. It was necessary to seclude him for a few hours, when he became tranquil, though he was not himself for some days afterwards. The mother, on visiting him, confirmed the previous history, and supplied the following additional and important facts: — The lad had always been passionate, and latterly he had become more so, when matters culminated in the acts previously described. She was sure he had never had an epileptic fit, though she fancied that one day after being in a passion he appeared somewhat faint and giddy. The father was a confirmed drunkard, and had run away to America two years ago. She herself acknowledged to habits of intemperance, and to bad health. She is small in stature and of unpleasing physiognomy. I was beginning to think of sending out this little fellow on a month's trial, and I mentioned my intention to the mother, but she was greatly alarmed at the prospect, and begged me to keep him a little longer. Luckily, I acceded to her request. A week afterwards, on February 13th, the boy became again excited, and had a distinct and severe epileptic seizure, from which he did not recover complete consciousness for some hours. The mask is hereby removed; that for which the rod and the treadmill were threatened before he came here now needs asylum supervision and care. Since the above date there has been no fit, no excitement, but a general improvement in health and physiognomy. How long am I to keep this young subject, and what is likely to be his future? I cannot tell. I have no doubt his disease has been conditioned by the antecedents of his parents, but I have much hope that under care and discipline he will stamp out his terrible inheritance and merge into a healthy and unfettered manhood. [Has since been discharged, recovered.]

In all cases which are included under Dr. Prichard's definition of moral insanity, it may be doubted whether, although there may be perfect freedom from delusions, there is not some disturbance of the intellectual faculties. Certainly in those which he has recorded, and which have been analyzed and commented upon by various authors, the intelligence does not appear to have been altogether normal, and in the majority delusions were subsequently developed. In children, more frequently than in adults, you find this moral insanity dissociated from serious intellectual derangement. A lad or a young girl will suddenly become depraved and vicious, lose all sense of decency, openly and defiantly commit self-abuse, destroy clothing, and perform acts which are the very antithesis of all which has been ever done before. Such cases, where the insane temperament is not marked or hereditary, are of hopeful prognosis; but, failing to improve, will become complicated by delusions and hallucinations. It is not improbable that the general erethistic condition, which is so often leagued with the insanity of early life, is as much dependent upon irritation of the spinal and sympathetic systems as upon centric disturbance of the cerebral hemispheres.

The moral insanity of later years is ordinarily associated with melancholia, and may or may not be complicated with suicidal impulses. A general change comes over the habits and inclinations. One previously remarkable for energy and decision will doubt and vacillate; slovenliness will take the place of order and cleanliness; little acts of impropriety will manifest themselves in one of previously unblemished life; he may become likewise reckless in his expenditure of money, though his antecedents have been those of thrift and economy. Subsequently the memory becomes impaired; there is more emotional disturbance and general incapacity; and a state of what is termed senile dementia precedes and ushers in the "dreariness and duskiness of age."

Dementia—Acute Primary; Chronic Primary; Secondary.

You will remember that I spoke to you on a former occasion of a derangement termed *Melancholia Attonita* or *Mélancolie avec Stupeur;* and I pointed out its diagnostic features from acute dementia. The latter disease now comes under our notice.

Although considered to be curable, acute primary dementia is a very alarming malady. The complete suspension of the faculties, the reduction from intelligence to the most abject passivity of automatic life, are of themselves startling even to the utter bewilderment of the lookers on. Moreover, the circumstance of its occurrence so frequently in the young, in whom we look for the highest manifestation of vital force and happiness, gives to it by contrast with our hopes and expectations a character of unmodified sadness. It is probable that in most cases of this nature there exists a previous instability and imperfection of nerve-element, which, though it may not have attracted notice by anything marked and special, is now retrospectively apprehended on the occasion of the sudden suspension of mental power. A very common cause of acute primary dementia is fright. I have a case now in the Asylum where fright resulting from the bite of a dog produced this shattering of the higher life and intelligence. The case is incurable, for epilepsy has supervened. An enormous responsibility attaches to those who terrify the young. A blow on the head, masturbation, fever, and the acute exanthematous diseases are concerned likewise in the factorship of this distressing malady. There is no doubt that the ear-boxing and head-thumping, once so practised at our schools, have laid the foundation of fatal cerebral mischief in a large number of cases. I once saw a lady who became suddenly and completely demented during convalescence from small-pox. She did not recover for eight months, and I feared that her case was hopeless. This derangement is incidental also to the puerperal state, as I shall have occasion to point out to you in another lecture. By sudden grief, or even sudden and ecstatic joy, is conditioned likewise this suspension of the moral and intelligential life. Pinel has recorded several instances, and I once knew a gentleman of large and robust frame who suddenly became oppressed to melancholy by the responsibility of a large fortune which had been unexpectedly left him, and then rapidly lapsed into a state of acute and confirmed dementia.

The symptoms of this disease are worthy of your attention. From one or other of the causes which I have above mentioned, you will find a previously intelligent youth or girl in a state of complete passivity. The countenance is blank and expressionless; the motor functions are ordinarily suspended, or, when existing, are of a monotonous and purposeless character. The calls of nature are unheeded—frequently the bladder has to be emptied artificially; food has in the same way to be administered by spoonfuls or the stomach-pump. The circulation is feeble, the temperature low, and there is general congestion of the venous system. Everything indicates want of vital energy and force. The patient will sit or stand with a vacant stare for weeks together; the perceptive and reflective faculties are alike suspended. He has to be dressed and undressed, and occasionally this is a process which he will resist, forming perhaps the only exception to a state of complete passivity. Sleep is not disturbed, as in the melancholia; and this forms one of the diagnostic signs between the two affections. Another diagnostic mark is the relaxed vacuity of expression, as compared with the utter gloom and moroseness and anxious physiognomy of melancholia—the former indicating what Guislain terms the "extinction," the latter the "oppression" of mental power. As a watch that has stopped from some unascertained cause will sometimes upon succussion resume for a few moments its ordinary movements, so these acutely demented subjects may occasionally be roused by shaking, or the action of a galvanic battery, into a momentary renewal of the intelligential life.

Acute dementia is not a common form of insanity, and when it takes place from a well-ascertained shock, in a constitution not otherwise materially impaired, the prognosis is decidedly favourable. But when by its approach the term primary is obviously not synonymous with acute dementia, there are frequently causes at work which forebode the most unpromising results. Self-abuse is of these the most pernicious and ineradicable. When to this is added the hereditary taint, so commonly ascertained to exist, chronic and complete dementia can be alone predicated as the issue.

The treatment of acute dementia is based upon well-recognised principles. Life is below par; we must bring it up to par. I often add quinine to the spoon-food, or to that which it is necessary to throw in by the stomach-pump—four or five grains twice a day; wine, warm clothing, friction, Turkish baths, occasional purgatives (aloetic), or an enema containing a teaspoonful of turpentine. A galvanic current transmitted through the spinal column morning and evening is decidedly beneficial. The cleanliness of these patients must be particularly attended to, the hairy parts being washed with carbolic acid soap, for vermin are quickly generated.

The recognition of chronic primary dementia in its earlier stages is not by any means easy, inasmuch as those who are obnoxious to it are very variable in their states and conditions. The stumbling memory and bewildered aspect of to-day may have changed into comparative retentiveness and intelligence to-morrow. There is an absence of delusions and hallucinations, and you naturally hesitate to stamp with incapacity those whose symptoms of fatuity have not yet become matured and permanent. I have a case now under observation of primary dementia which has been coming on for the last six months. The patient is utterly bewildered at times: he has no memory; he picks pockets, and, unconscious of the habit, wonders, when taxed with having certain articles which do not belong to him, how they came into his possession. At other times he is comparatively bright and intelligent. Probably the brain-cells are undergoing a process of atrophic degeneration known as " white softening."

Many men after an active life, in which the faculties have been unduly strained, or sensuality inordinately indulged in, gradually evidence enfeeblement of thought and judgment, strangely contrasting with their former vigour and capacity, and fall step by step into "second childishness and mere oblivion." There may have been complete freedom from maniacal or melancholic symptoms. The failure of memory, especially for recent occurrences, is one of the earliest symptoms of approaching mental decay; or an apoplectic attack, with temporary hemiplegia or loss of speech, may precede the mental symptoms. Such cases are very hopeless, though certainly at times a very marked and inexplicable (though temporary) improvement takes place when least expected and not at all prognosticated.

The subsidence of the various forms of acute insanity which have been brought under your notice, when not resulting in recovery or in death, is transmuted into secondary dementia as its almost inevitable tomb. There the pride and splendour of the intellectual life are ended, and upon its portals is written no "*Resurgam*." Considerably more than half the cases which fill our asylums are "compounded of the remains" and effects of antecedent maladies. And the forms assumed by the "shattered wrecks of mental organization," which make up the aggregate of consecutive dementia, are endless in variety of detail, and constitute an interesting study in walking the wards of a large asylum. In some there is a quiet and orderly passivity, which, though associated with delusions, finds no outward expression, as under those acute ideational disturbances which once rioted here, and have now made shipwreck of the supreme centre of intelligence. These subjects will state their delusions when under pressure, and affirm the reality of their convictions with a temporary and emotional excitement; but you perceive they lack the intensity which they once possessed, and are babbled out with a childish reiteration contrasting strangely with the fervour and sparkle of earlier days. "The paths of mental association," as Dr. Maudsley expresses it, "are broken up, so that the delusions are cut off from any active influence upon such mental functions as are left, and all real interest in the past or present is abolished."

The actions and attitudes of many dements and chronic maniacs are singularly grotesque and amusing; so also are the modes of personal decoration and adornment. They almost equal in variety of shape and colour the uncertificated daughters of the folly which bears the name of Fashion, and the Fair which is labelled Vanity. In looking into the airing-courts of an asylum you may see geometrical figures which have been paced into shape by the daily treadings of these monotonous movers. Some walk in circles, some in straight lines, some in rhomboids. Some lie on the ground, having lost all energy, manifesting nothing but the listlessness of life. Some always sit in the same corners, stand in the same places and positions, with closed eyes and expressionless faces. Others are more demonstrative, dancing and singing, gesticulating, shouting, tearing their clothes, or stripping themselves naked. Some are engaged in top-like gyrations, others in somersaults, or in fantastic muscular displays worthy of those young Arabs of the pavement who invite by their revolutions the loose halfpence of thoughtless passers-by. And these are not the extremes of that degraded condition to which these miserable creatures are ultimately reduced. There is a lower stage, in which the calls of nature are unheeded; they eat and drink their own excretions; swallow glass, rags, crockery, rubbish of any kind. In a patient who died last year I found in the stomach 9 lbs. of rubbish, chiefly consisting of pieces of cloth, stones, and bits of crockery and tobacco-pipe.

There is nothing to do in these cases but to watch them carefully, bathe, and change their linen frequently; try to establish periodicity of function, by taking them to the closet at fixed times. Much is to be done in this way; but even then their last years of life—or rather existence, for such a condition is unworthy of the name of life—are filthy and degrading to an extent which cannot be realized by any but those who are familiar with what we call the "dirty" wards of an asylum.

LECTURE V.

Puerperal Insanity.

You will remember my having told you, when speaking of the difficulty of classifying mental diseases, that I thought some modern writers had done much more to embarrass than to simplify. The *impedimenta* which certain persons like to throw in the way of nosological simplicity are truly astounding. They constitute what Guislain well calls "un bagage symptomalogique," which even the best memory finds it difficult to carry.

The presumed causes of insanity do not furnish distinguishing characteristics sufficient to justify a causal classification. Alluding to this important matter Dr. Sankey truly says, "Insanity occurring in a phthisical person may be in some way modified in its course, progress, and, perhaps, phenomena. It would be strange, indeed, were it not so, for even a fracture of the leg may be modified in its progress of recovery by the existence of phthisis or other disease. But we should not think of speaking of phthisical fractures or scrofulous broken legs. I would not attempt to deny that phthisis, the puerperal condition, scrofula, syphilis, congenital organization, and that which is called hereditary predisposition may all act as disturbing causes to the regular development or progress of the mental symptoms. But there is no ground, any the more, for asserting that the disease in these patients is different in species; and nothing is gained, but, on the contrary, much confusion arises, from the multiplication of the so-called varieties of insanity."

Excepting only that form of alienation which is incidental to the puerperal state, I most entirely endorse these remarks. Even to that state, indeed, they may in strict accuracy be applied; for Dr. Gooch himself has said, " If a physician were taken into the chamber of a patient whose mind had become disordered from lying-in or nursing, he could not tell from the mere condition of her mind that the disease had originated from these causes." And Dr. J. Thompson Dickson, formerly resident medical officer at St. Luke's Hospital, in an instructive contribution to the study of this subject, published in the *Journal of Mental Science*, affirms— " In almost all instances, perhaps in all, there is a potentiality of insanity, either from hereditary transmission or specially and accidentally induced, but not associated with the parturient condition. It seems highly probable, though the evidence on this point is as yet incomplete, that without the potentiality above spoken of, a patient will not become insane as a consequence of parturition; and it appears to be much more correct to speak of the cases as insanity appearing at the puerperal season, than to use the term 'puerperal' in an adjectival sense, as though the insanity was a special form peculiar to child-bearing."

But considering how frequently practitioners are called upon to treat cases of puerperal, who do not see, or seldom see, other forms of insanity, I regard it as a matter of importance to give you a distinct account of this distressing malady; for I do not know anything more alarming to a family circle, or more trying to their medical attendant. All that seemed so bright and cheering has suddenly become changed. With the new life had been expected the new joy; and there has come the unmeasured tribulation.

Puerperal insanity may assume either the form of mania, melancholia, or dementia; and it may occur at three distinct periods: 1st. During the process of utero-gestation. 2nd. Immediately or shortly after labour. 3rd. At a much later period, during and from the exhausting effects of lactation. Mania is more frequent than melancholia, and seems chiefly to attach itself to the second period; melancholia belongs rather to the first and third periods; dementia is common to the last two. But I think it is beyond a doubt that many of the cases assuming both the melancholic and the maniacal type, in the puerperal condition, have a tendency to fuse themselves, as it were, with acute dementia. An excitement of days may succeed or precede a period of the most distressing and abject passivity. There does not appear to be any evidence to show that the insanity of utero-gestation is in any way dependent upon that condition, or has any causal relation thereto. It is a mere empirical coincidence, and is not likely to be benefited by the induction of premature labour. In two private cases which I saw of this form, the insanity was of the maniacal type, and was distinctly hereditary. In one of them the maniacal symptoms never abated, and after ceaseless and incoherent chattering for five months the patient died. In the other the symptoms were modified during the period of labour; but there was a subsequent recurrence of them, and the patient became the subject of chronic mania, and a permanent inmate of a private asylum.

At the time, I repeat, when the body is sustaining the effects of labour, the maniacal type of mental disturbance is most frequent. It is more dangerous to life, but less dangerous to reason, than the melancholic, which appertains rather to that period when the system is debilitated by nursing.

An illustration of each, drawn from life by a master-hand, will serve you better than a general description, for (as Dr. Gooch truly says) "such descriptions are commonly formed of a bewildering multiplicity of circumstances, which never occurred together in one and the same instance, so that they are pictures which resemble nothing in nature—like the abstract ideas of the old physicians."

"A lady, who, I was told, had had a 'brain fever' after her former lying-in, came to London to be attended by me in her next confinement, and took a furnished house in a street near Cavendish Square. She had a short and easy labour, a good supply of milk, nursed her child, and continued to do well for so many days that her friends concluded all danger was over. Nevertheless, from the circumstances of her former confinement, I visited her twice a day, but I detected nothing which indicated the approach of disease. Her pulse was not quick, her nights were disturbed only by occasionally suckling the child, and her manner and appearance were unaltered. On the tenth day after her delivery the shop of a pianoforte maker in Oxford Street caught fire. This occasioned a great bustle in the neighbourhood; but, as her sitting-room did not look into the street, it was kept from her knowledge during the day; but in the evening, while she was standing at her window, which looked into a yard at the back of the house, a piece of burning matter fell within her sight. I saw her about two hours afterwards, at nine in the evening: she was not herself; her manner was agitated. On being questioned about her feelings she kept silent for some time, and then answered abruptly. Her pulse was quick, and her look and manner odd and unnatural. I slept in the house. At four o'clock in the morning the nurse awaked me, and said that her mistress had had no sleep; that she was sitting up in bed talking to herself, but that instant had expressed a wish to see me. I rose and went to her. There was only a rush-light in a remote part of the chamber. As soon as she saw who I was she told me to sit down and look at her. I said, 'I do.' 'What do you see?' 'Nothing but yourself.' 'Look at my head.' 'I do.' 'Do you see nothing particular there?' 'Nothing.' 'Then I was presumptuous. I thought that a glorious light came to my temples and shone about my head. I thought I was the Virgin Mary.' It is curious that the immediate cause of the disturbance was a lighted body, and that the first hallucination was concerned about light. She was put under the care of a nurse accustomed to such patients, and an eminent physician saw her with me. Her pulse was soft, and never very quick, and her face pale. Nevertheless, from a fear of congestion in the brain her head was shaved, and ten ounces of blood were extracted from the scalp by cupping-glasses, without diminishing in the slightest degree her violence and incoherence. Her conjunctivæ were yellow, her tongue furred, and her bowels costive. Hence she was moderately purged; and about three weeks from the commencement of the illness she returned to her country seat well. She was confined again about fifteen months afterwards, without any recurrence of the disease. About a week before this latter delivery she had the jaundice, of which she was cured by calomel and aloetic purgatives before she fell in labour. It is practically important to notice that she had the jaundice at the time of her first confinement, and became maniacal; that she had a slight degree of it during her second confinement, and suffered the same disease; that she was completely jaundiced before her third confinement; that it was removed by purgatives before labour, and that she this time escaped her mental derangement."

You will observe that the treatment of Dr. Gooch's day was that of depletion. I do not know what would be thought of anyone who now resorted to cupping-glasses to the scalp, under fear of congestion, where brains are singularly bloodless, and of "paraphrenitis" without headache and intolerance of light. This unfortunate lady recovered, in spite of the blood-letting to which she was subjected. The experience of the learned physician, from whose note-book the above case is taken, led him to see the evils of lowering the vital forces of child-bearing women even under the most intense maniacal excitement. "Cerebral excitement," he writes, "is often aggravated by depletion, and in some cases, as I shall have occasion to relate, absolutely brought on by it."

The only other criticism which I feel called upon to make respecting the graphic picture of puerperal mania which I have shown to you, is upon the expressed curiousness of its author that the immediate cause of the disturbance and the first hallucination were equally referable to a lighted body. This is just what might have been expected, and indicates most forcibly the highly erethistic condition of the sensorium, and its consequent inability to rid itself of the luminous impression made upon it during the first acute stage of disease.

The melancholia which attaches itself to a period some five or six months after labour, has been attributed by certain writers to the discontinuance of nursing on the part of the mother. But there is no evidence to support this view, and it is entirely opposed to the experience of Dr. Gooch. The symptoms of debility preceding and necessitating the act of weaning clearly point to lactation, in constitutions previously impaired and feeble, as the causal phenomenon. An immense number of women moving in the upper circles of society can spare no time from the allurements of indolent and voluptuous life, for the performance of those functions which are the natural sequence and outcome of the utero-gestative process. But nature is kind and indulgent; and they do not suffer from the forced suppression and neglect of what is commonly regarded as a mammalian privilege.

"I must have known this done [the milk suppressed] in more than a hundred instances during the first week after delivery,—a time much more liable to the disordered mind than a later period,— and in not one did it occasion puerperal insanity. In all the cases which I have seen months after delivery the weaning has been the consequence of the disease, not the disease the consequence of the weaning. The patients had been reduced in health by nursing, their memories had become enfeebled, their spirits depressed, and their minds ultimately disordered; and they were directed to wean their children because they had neither milk nor strength to enable them to nurse." So writes Dr. Gooch. He further alludes to the melancholia resulting from the debilitating effects of nursing, by pointing out a peculiarity in the commencement of the disease which is seldom or never noticed at the commencement of mania—viz., an incipient stage in which the mind is wrong, but right enough to recognise the fact of its aberration. This, I take it, is to be explained by the fact that, there being no ideal exaltation and disturbance of the comparing faculties, the mind is able, under the slower and more measured processes of its disorganization, to feel and discern its impending danger.

One of the most painful features of that class of diseases which we are now discussing is the dislike so frequently manifested by the patient towards her nearest relatives and friends. She suspects, and hates, and has horrible delusions as to her husband's and even her own fidelity. These are they which generate suicidal impulses. Frequently they are long and persistent, and accompanied by the most distressing expressions of contrition and the most harrowing sense of self-humiliation. Under these circumstances you will easily understand how the bringing together again of one who stands in this relationship to the sufferer and herself is often a very hazardous proceeding during the earliest stage of convalescence, and one requiring the greatest care and discrimination. I have in my mind's eye a very painful instance of an imprudence of this kind, where the importunity—nay, the insistence—of the husband produced the most disastrous results.

But, naturally enough, a husband and his children are intensely anxious to see the object of their affections at the earliest possible moment, and the physician finds it difficult to resist the importunities which beset him. Firmness, however, on your parts, and enforced separation, must be maintained until the patient herself gives some evidence of a desire for the renewal of family intercourse. The expressed desire is the first indication of its need, and a tacit acknowledgment that the previous suspicions were real delusions.

At times an intense desire to commit suicide is associated with the melancholic type of puerperal insanity, and is one of the earliest evidences of its existence. I remember a case in which a lady who had been confined about six weeks, and whose nurse (being an old favourite in the family) had not yet left her, nearly succeeded in hanging herself. She had had a good labour, and, though a weak and rather delicate person, was nursing her child bravely and nutritiously. I had seen her in the morning, and the only change in her condition which I had noticed was that she stared at me unusually, and said she had not slept well the previous night. This statement was confirmed by the nurse. As I intended seeing her again in the evening I did not leave any instructions about an opiate, but the bowels being costive I ordered a dose of castor oil. My patient had dined early with the nurse. They were sitting together by the fire afterwards, and the latter had dropped asleep with the baby in her lap. But the sleeper was suddenly roused up by the noise of something falling, and immediately discovered that her mistress had suspended herself to a brass hook by one of her garters and a pocket-handkerchief tied together. The garter had fortunately given way, and the fall had disclosed the tragedy which was all but consummated. For three weeks this lady remained in a state of profound melancholia, and there was the greatest difficulty in getting her to take food. But she ultimately recovered and did well, and passed through two subsequent labours without any untoward symptoms.

Occasionally the alienation of the puerperal state assumes the form of acute dementia, a sudden shock to the nervous system being the immediate cause.

But, as I before mentioned, many of the maniacal and melancholic cases associated with the puerperal state appear to be on the border-line of suspended faculties. A case was narrated to me some years ago of a poor woman who had been confined about ten days, and was progressing satisfactorily. Her husband was struck by lightning, and she saw him brought into the house dead. She gave a wild shriek, and fell to the ground. To the woman the moral shock was more disastrous than the physical shock to the man, for she remained a lunatic for life.

There is also a form of mental disturbance, of which I have seen one instance, and of which Dr. Gooch gives a very striking example. It appertains to the neurotic temperament, and may be termed cataleptoid dementia. A nervous lady, twenty-nine years of age, had been often pregnant, but had only borne one living child. After delivery, at the seventh month, of a dead fœtus, she was seized with a violent left hemicranial neuralgia, intense flatulence of stomach, and great depression of spirits. She told her husband she had been unfaithful, and tried to cut her throat the next morning. Her violence became intense, and she was put under the care of a regular attendant, and confined with a strait-waistcoat. Drs. Gooch and Sutherland visited her. "A few days," says the former, "after our first visit we were summoned to observe a remarkable change in her symptoms. The attendants said she was dying or in a trance. She was lying in bed motionless, and apparently senseless. It had been said that the pupils were dilated and motionless, and some apprehension of effusion on the brain had been entertained; but on coming to examine them closely, it was found that they readily contracted when the light fell upon them. Her eyes were open, but no rising of the chest, no movement of the nostrils, no appearance of respiration, could be seen. The only signs of life were her warmth and pulse; the latter was, as we had hitherto observed it, weak, and about 120. Her fæces and urine were voided in bed. The trunk of the body was now lifted so as to form rather an obtuse angle with the limbs (a most uncomfortable posture), and there left with nothing to support it. There she continued sitting while we were asking questions and conversing, so that many minutes must have passed. One arm was now raised, then the other, and where they were left there they remained. It was now a curious sight to see her sitting up in bed, her eyes open, staring lifelessly, her arms outstretched, yet without any visible sign of animation. She was very thin and pallid, and looked like a corpse that had been propped up, and had stiffened in this attitude. We now took her out of bed, placed her upright, and endeavoured to rouse her by calling loudly in her ears, but in vain. She stood up, but as inanimate as a statue; the slightest push put her off her balance; no exertion was made to regain it;

she would have fallen if I had not caught her. She went into this state three several times; the first time it lasted fourteen hours, the second time twelve hours, and the third time nine hours, with waking intervals of two days after the first fit, and one day after the second. After this the disease resumed the ordinary form of melancholia, and three months from the time of her delivery she was well enough to resume her domestic duties." Dr. Sutherland has mentioned several similar but more prolonged cases.

These, then, are the forms of puerperal insanity which you will meet with in practice. What is their danger to life? What to reason? What is likely to be their probable duration? And what is the treatment indicated? Now, I should tell you that the statistics of public asylums furnish us with but very meagre and unreliable evidence concerning puerperal insanity; for the disease bearing that name is one chiefly of *home* and *private* treatment. Moreover, it is one to which, like the gout, the rich are more obnoxious than the poor. The large lying-in hospitals of Dublin and London do not yield many instances of that mental disturbance, which, coming at the season of parturition, or during the progress of nursing, so alarms and terrifies. The cases which are taken to public asylums are not of this class. They consist, rather, of broken-down persons who have been unsuccessfully treated outside, and are at the time of admission in an advanced stage of debility and disease. Often they are those who have been insane before, and who are weighted with the terrible heritage of an ancestral taint. There is a natural and well-justified indisposition on the part of medical practitioners to send the acute forms of puerperal insanity to asylums; for recovery is sometimes very rapid, and the character of a person is in one sense really injured by confinement in a madhouse. It is a blot upon the family escutcheon. So that you may get into sad trouble with your patient's friends if you subject to asylum restraint and discipline a case which has a quickly successful issue.

It is only when your patient becomes very violent and unmanageable, or has very determined suicidal tendencies, that you are justified in placing her in confinement.

In respect of their danger to life, Dr. Gooch states that in his day there was a very common belief among medical men of great general eminence, but small special experience, that the diseases of this class were never fatal. "Whilst I was attending," he writes, "the near relation of one of the most eminent and experienced of the provincial practitioners of this island, a letter arrived from him, begging the family to have no fears—that he had seen many such cases during his long life, and never saw one die; and even the late Dr. Baillie, when consulted about a case, remarked that 'the question was not *whether* she was to get well, but *when* she was to get well.' The latter patient died within a week after this prognosis." The real fact is that a very large proportion of cases of puerperal insanity recover; it is one of the most curable forms of mental alienation. Death is very unusual, and probably only takes place in those rare cases of the maniacal type, where the excitement begins soon after delivery, and there is a steady maintenance of quick pulse and high temperature. We then write down "maniacal exhaustion" as the immediate cause. Drs. William Hunter and Gooch allude to this form as involving great danger to life, and add that when "blood-letting" is employed a fatal issue is inevitable. And the latter physician affirms, in reference to the curability of puerperal insanity, "Of the patients about whom I have been consulted, I know only two who are now, after many years, disordered in mind, and of them one had already been so before her marriage." It is important to bear in mind that he is speaking chiefly, if not entirely, of the upper classes of society, among whom his practice was very extensive. Anyhow, he clearly thinks that the information to be gathered from tables which have hitherto been published by various authors is "unnecessarily gloomy and discouraging."

Dr. Conolly says, "In private practice I cannot myself recollect one case of puerperal insanity which did not terminate favourably, and in the majority of cases recovery took place in from four to seven months." "The appearance of levity, childishness, and imbecility in some cases of puerperal insanity discourages the practitioner, but in reality these symptoms are but temporary, and the patient generally recovers."

Repeating, then, my previous assertion that asylum statistics are not to be relied on respecting the insanity of child-bearing women, inasmuch as they take no account of acute cases or of any of short duration, it may be stated that the maniacal form is recovered from most quickly, although during its existence it is more dangerous to life than the melancholic type. The latter is more likely to be prolonged and permanent, and it attaches itself chiefly to the later period — the period of lactation.

My own experience of puerperal insanity is very limited, but from what I can gather I should say nine out of ten get well under twelve months; that quite half the cases get well under six months; and that, where there is no hereditary taint, the recurrence of insanity in a subsequent labour is very improbable. But, obviously, great care and circumspection should be exercised both by the friends and the medical attendant in every case where it is known that madness of any form has been a previous condition of either the utero-gestative or parturient period. One thing is quite certain (and my friend, Dr. Monro, of St. Luke's Hospital, confirms me in the opinion), that in no form more

K

than in that of puerperal insanity is it so necessary to be constantly on our guard against surprises and misadventures. The life of the child or of the mother herself may be sacrificed by a little carelessness on the part of the attendants in charge. These remarks are specially applicable to melancholia associated with delusions or hallucinations.

The treatment of puerperal, like that of all other forms of insanity, has a twofold relation: on the one hand to therapeutic agents, on the other to dietetics and general management.

No one can study the graphic pictures drawn by Dr. Gooch without perceiving the fatal evils of blood-letting and lowering treatment generally. And no one can reflect upon that "peculiarity of nerve and of mind which distinguishes the female from the male constitution," without coming to the conclusion that sleep and nourishment are the great things needed to restore that healthy organization, the departure from which has conditioned so great functional disturbance. Be assured that there is nothing to fear from what Sydenham terms "too great spirituousness and richness of the blood." Its thinness and "vapidity," however, may well alarm us.

It is of great importance to begin your attack upon this disease by thoroughly cleansing the bowels with a good aloetic purge; for commonly there is a foul and coated tongue, with offensive breath, and constipation. Sometimes there are prodigious and highly fetid accumulations of fæcal matter in the lower bowels, the removal of which acts like a charm. I know not how it is, but so it is, that the least interesting of our visceral territories —known as the rectum—does contain vaster mines of that which may fertilize the soil when bounded anteriorly by a uterus than when fronted with spermatic cords. A most instructive case illustrative of this is narrated by Dr. Gooch. You must next endeavour to procure sleep, and your hypnotics of whatever kind are much more likely to be efficacious if you have adopted the preliminary measure above indicated. Where there are the means of using it, and there is no extreme violence and resistance on the part of your patient, a warm bath may be of great service. Its soothing effects are sometimes very marked. You may give your sedative, with liquid nourishment, at once, and it will probably be just flooding the tender brain-cells with delicious calm as you remove the sufferer from the bath to her bed. Formerly, as you know, the hypnotic resorted to was opium — probably Battley's solution. An excellent preparation was (and still is) a solution of the bimeconate of morphia, prepared by Mr. Squire, of Oxford Street. But all these remedies are, as it seems to me, dwarfed into insignificance by the giant hydrate of chloral—in every sense a more satisfactory remedy. It not only is more certain to produce sleep, but it is more certain to leave fewer unpleasant after-effects. It does not produce headache; it does not constipate the bowels; it does not impair the digestion and produce nausea—one or all of which are well recognised and frequent sequelæ of opium. Indeed, opium has been vastly overrated in the treatment of insanity generally. Begin by a dose of half a drachm, and repeat it in four hours if necessary. Nourishment must be abundant and frequent, for the circulation is always feeble, and the tendency to exhaustion great. Liebig's extract of meat, beaten up with eggs, milk, and wine or brandy, constitutes an excellent compound. Do not hesitate, if your patient has a craving for it, to let her have a mutton chop and a glass of stout. In fact, the expressed desire for food indicates more than anything else its necessity.

If these remedies fail to produce satisfactory results, and your patient continues violent and unmanageable, you must have two special attendants to watch her; and they must be careful that no knives and forks, or destructive instruments of any kind, are left lying about the room. They must be equally careful about securing the chamber windows, and never leaving their charge alone. A neglect of this rule may involve, and has involved, the most dire catastrophes. Removal from town to the country is often a most desirable and salutary measure. There are but few cases occurring among the upper classes that cannot be managed in this way, because money will buy skilled and trained attendants, the best medical advice, and enable you to convert a private residence into a temporary asylum. With the lower orders it is, of course, otherwise, and you must send your patient to the institution which the law provides for her relief and maintenance. It is of importance that the child should be at once weaned, both on its own account, and on account of the mother. The drink that is drained from the fountain of mad breasts can contain but few desirable elements. You have nothing to fear from the suppression of milk; you have everything to fear from that which tends to produce exhaustion and debility. The mammæ, if at all full for a few days, are easily managed. When the mental disturbance commences a few days after delivery, there is sometimes a premature suppression of the lochial discharge. You must try and set it free by the application of a turpentine stupe to the abdomen. In this you will be aided by your general treatment.

As the acute symptoms subside, the tendency still not being towards recovery, but rather towards that chronic condition of abnormal intelligence and feeling which may obtain for many months, you must be careful to bring into play all the curative weapons of your therapeutic, dietetic, and hygienic armoury. These are abundant air, exercise, bathing, generous living, with moderate and well-adjusted stimulants. Keep the head cool; the heart, stomach, and feet warm. Enforce your rules with the wayward and wilful; persuade the gentle and timid. In no case is perseverance so necessary, and ultimately so well rewarded. You must continue the hypnotics at night, if necessary, and you may vary the chloral hydrate with two or three drachms of the hemlock juice of the British Pharmacopœia. These are better than opium; the best preparation of which, however, is the bimeconate of morphia before mentioned. As the nights improve, and the sleep gets more natural, you may gradually discontinue — that is, by decreasing doses — the therapeutic agents by which you have hitherto invited it. But do not omit at any time the warm night stimulant, with liquid nutriment. I give all my sleepless and invalid patients a basin of brandy and sago at bedtime. It is a narcotic which *invites* but does not *force* sleep. In treating the melancholic type of puerperal insanity, you must observe the same rules, being more on your guard against suicide. Here, too, there is more frequent difficulty about food, the patient sometimes obstinately refusing it, under the delusion that it contains poison, or that she is ordered not to take it. But the melancholic will often refuse food because they cannot energize themselves into the act of feeding. They lie in a state of complete passivity, and are indifferent to all about them. But a careful and attentive nurse will manage to get down by spoonfuls a great deal of nourishment in the twenty-four hours. Do not forget to ascertain daily about the condition of the bladder, and remember that its leakage does not necessarily imply its emptiness. The general instructions which I before gave you as to artificial feeding and hypodermic injection will here equally serve you, if necessary.

Of so much importance is it, that I must again make allusion, before I conclude this lecture, to the question of forced separation from your patient of her husband and children. One of the saddest features of these cases is the morbid hatred which usurps for awhile the natural home of affection and love. You must yield to it, and not combat it. It is useless to argue with those whose instinctive life is so perverted and disturbed. Dr. Gooch thus puts the matter: "Interviews with relations and friends are commonly passed in increased emotion, remonstrance, altercation, and obviously do harm. Large experience also is decidedly favourable to separation as a general rule; yet there may be exceptions which the intelligent practitioner will detect by observing the effect of intercourse. The husband ought never to be left alone with his deranged wife, for obvious reasons. I have known more than once a neglect of this rule produce consequences which left in the minds of those concerned a never-ending regret."

Remember this, then, and therewith the equally important circumstance that it may occasionally be desirable to make tentative efforts at renewed intercourse. It is quite possible, from fear of re-creating the delusions which enforced separation, that you may unreasonably prolong it.

There are no cases requiring such a combined exercise of patience, and skill, and tact, and delicacy of handling, as cases of puerperal insanity. And there are no cases, therefore, which afford you afterwards such a retrospect of pleasure and satisfaction if you have managed to bring them to a successful issue.

LECTURE VI.

General Paralysis of the Insane.

I PROPOSE to speak to you to-day of a disease which, considering its frequency, is less observed and recognised by those who have not made insanity a special study, than any other to which the human family is obnoxious. Although there can be no doubt of its antiquity, even alienist physicians had not described it as a distinct pathological state until the beginning of the present century. Haslam saw it imperfectly; Esquirol, Delaye, and Bayle recognised it; and Calmeil subsequently, in 1826, pourtrayed its distinctive features in a monograph, which drew to the malady the attention of our own Conolly.

It must not, I repeat, be regarded as

"A new disease unknown to men;"

for Shakespeare, as my friend Dr. Shaw has pointed out, grasped it with his comprehensive mind, when he puts into the mouth of Ulysses (*Troilus and Cressida*, Act II., Scene iii.) the following language:—

> "Things small as nothing, for request's sake only,
> He makes important; possessed he is with greatness,
> And speaks not to himself, but with a pride
> That quarrels at self breadth. Imagin'd worth
> Holds in his blood such swoll'n and hot disease,
> That, 'twixt his mental and his active parts,
> Kingdom'd Achilles in promotion rages,
> And batters down himself. What should I say ?—
> He is so plaguy proud that the death tokens of it
> Cry ' No recovery.' "

Now, it is fair to assume that our great dramatist intended in this passage to attribute to the son of Peleus a state of mental derangement with which his experienced eye had brought him in contact, but which no leech of his time had, to our knowledge, shaped into a distinct and morbid entity. And certainly it is an accurate and truthful description of the disease now under consideration.

It is of great importance, in the first place, that you should recognise it in its early stage, for, as I said before, the disease is very common, and on the increase, and furnishes sufficiently defined landmarks to those who will take the trouble to look out for them. And yet it is certain that there are received every year into our asylums a large number of cases, certified by well-educated members of the profession to be uncomplicated with paralysis, which we are able at a glance to pronounce as hopeless by reason of this complication.

There should be no difficulty really in recognising these physical symptoms, though before their appearance it is easy to understand that the earliest evidence of ideational derangement should only be appreciated by those who are specially familiar with its diagnostic value. For myself, I have come to the conclusion that very frequently the first scene of the three-act tragedy of this disease is played in a police-court to a vulgar and indiscriminating audience. I have many times noted this in the daily reports of metropolitan vagabondage, and prophesied too truly the eventful drama unfolding itself in Worship Street or Westminster would, within the walls of Colney Hatch Asylum, be brought to its sad and disastrous close. For (to preserve the metaphor) the tragedy of general paralysis is, with few exceptions, one of three acts full of varied incident, of which the order of interest is inverted; for it culminates in the first and second, and is altogether absent from the last. With these three acts, or stages, it will be my endeavour to make you acquainted.

One modern author, Dr. Sankey (formerly one of the medical superintendents at Hanwell), is so impressed with the prominence of the incidents in the second act, that in his description of this malady he gives it precedence over the first. But this appears to me so strange a proceeding that I shall not follow it, but rather place matters before you as Nature represents them, in legitimate order and sequence. And this is the more necessary because, as Dr. Wilks and other authors have pointed out, there is a form of general paralysis simulating in all respects the disease of that name associated with insanity, except in the occurrence of maniacal excitement and grandiose delusions. Certainly many cases of this kind are met with in asylum practice, and they constitute for the more part the exceptions before alluded to of the triple arrangement of symptomatic phenomena. These latter cases are likewise on the increase, and the London hospitals contain many illustrations of what is termed "progressive paralysis," in which no insanity has evidenced itself. There is probably defective memory and power of apprehension, inability to compare and to associate; but these things do not constitute that startling malady whose varied incidents I am about to describe to you.

The first or incubatory stage of general paralysis of the insane consists of those prodromata which alike characterize so commonly the initiatory period of mania or melancholia. There is an alteration in the habits of the individual, slight and scarcely noticeable at first, but soon acquiring a prominence which attracts the attention of all who are brought in contact with him. A few days of depression are not infrequent. He has not the same interest in his business or profession. He has larger views and a loftier ambition. He appears to do everything eagerly and in a hurry, and so he does nothing well. He complains at times of pain in the head, and he is liable to violent outbursts of passion if he is in any way thwarted. "Pinhole pupils," as we term them, are not an infrequent accompaniment of this stage, and one pupil is constantly larger than the other, becoming more marked as the disease progresses.

This symptom has been held by some writers to be diagnostic of the disease under consideration; but my experience will not confirm this opinion, for I am persuaded that unequal dilatation frequently obtains in other forms of insanity. Matters now become more marked and complicated. There is absence from home, unmindfulness of the family ties, a forgetfulness of engagements, an indifference to order, and method, and punctuality. There is, so to speak, a general untidiness of mind, and the whole life becomes inconsistent with its antecedents. "Fastness" and "loudness" (two slang but comprehensive terms) may now express the general condition of one to whose nature, perhaps, such elements have heretofore been altogether foreign. There may or may not at this period be a slight thickness of speech, and a want of harmonious facial expression.

The second act may be summarized as an aggravation and development of all the phenomena of the first, with other and more significant readings. The "fastness" is evidenced alike in language and in acts, and eventuates in a recklessness of conduct which is truly alarming. Money is scattered freely and indiscriminately upon anyone and everybody, whether friend or stranger. New projects now unfold themselves; impossible schemes are concocted; fresh and foolish ideas are generated from day to day; money disbursements are made upon a scale previously unknown, and upon utterly unworthy objects. You have had pointed out to you before the absurdity and extravagances of some of the delusions of the insane, but you will note in this disease not only their extravagance and grandeur, but their utter absurdity and foolishness. In illustration of this I may mention the case of a clergyman of ample means and exemplary character, who came to London for a week, put up at a first-class hotel, and commenced his lively career there by bringing in at night three women of the town. His indignation was greatly aroused when the landlord refused to let them pass beyond the hall. The next day he purchased at different shops four pianos, all of which he ordered to be sent to his rooms. The proprietor became alarmed, obtained with difficulty the address of his friends in the country, and telegraphed to them immediately of these strange proceedings. I saw this gentleman the following afternoon, and pronounced him to be hopelessly insane—the subject of general paralysis. His pupils were unequal, his articulation was imperfect, his breath characteristically offensive. He died in less than twelve months, in one of the epileptiform seizures so common in the course of this malady. There was nothing to do but to place this patient in an asylum at once. He would have bought up half London in a week, had crowds round him in the streets daily, and given the police and magistrates an infinity of labour. His indignation at the idea of any restraint upon his freedom, and his subsequent violence, were very marked. I think I cannot do better than give you an extract from an excellent monograph on this disease by Dr. Skae, of Edinburgh, who thus describes the foolish and extravagant ideas, to which the French have given the term *délire ambitieux :*—

"The patient fancies that he is possessed of enormous wealth; he is full of projects for the benefit of mankind; he is about to purchase and endow libraries and churches for the public good. He is a prince ennobled by the Queen, about to marry a Spanish countess; he is possessed of fleets laden with gold and diamonds. The house in which he lives is a palace; all the attendants and females are his lords and ladies; the walls are gilded, the windows are made of diamonds; he himself made the sun which illuminates them; he is a mighty conqueror, and destroyed Sebastopol, captured the Emperor of Russia, but graciously pardoned him; he is God himself, and wields universal and omnipotent power. He can talk in any language; he can sing (and he does sing readily, but most discordantly); he can write most beautiful novels and enchanting poetry. He has carriages and horses without number—steamboats waiting to convey him to London to see the Queen—schemes of universal conquest or universal philanthropy. In the midst of all this imaginary power and grandeur, he is (and this is a very characteristic feature of general paralysis, as compared with other forms of insanity with similar delusions) docile and facile; he is diverted from the highest enterprise or the most important duty by the simplest request; he forgets the conquest of Europe, or the immediate commands of her Majesty, for a walk round the airing-ground with an imbecile companion, to whom he talks condescendingly, promising him a dukedom or a bishopric. Everything about him is good—everyone is so kind—his food is first-rate; he offers a cheque for £75,000 for the purchase of the asylum, and promises to endow it with unbounded munificence, and to convert it into a paradise of brilliancy and bliss."

It is very noticeable in this disastrous malady that the patient rushes from one absurd fancy to another, there being an absence of that fixity of delusion so common in ordinary mania or melancholia. He will assent to any absurd proposition which you may make to him, undertake any achievement, however gigantic; embark in any speculation, however ridiculous, with a sanguineness which is characteristic of the disease (with rare exceptions) up to the last glimmer of his mental faculties. This sanguineness is so remarkable as to tinge and colour the whole temperament under conditions and circumstances of the most distressing physical nature.

I have a patient now, a general paralytic, near the end of his chequered career, with large ulcers on his legs; but his legs are made of gold. He is the Emperor of the world, and I am his lieutenant-general in command. He is literally insensible to pain (and this anæsthesia is very remarkable in some cases), and, being questioned as to his condition, describes himself as "first-rate." This expression, indeed, is so common in general paralysis, that I have come to regard it as almost pathognomonic—the verbal formula of a hopeless malady. No happiness which you or I shall ever feel—such is the irony of disease!—can approach the supremacy of pleasure and satisfaction which belongs to him who is the subject of this most dire affliction. In one sense, it is a compensation to see the patient himself so utterly unconscious of his physical degradation; and yet it is sufficiently humiliating to behold the gradual descent of the moral and material ladder—the importation of theft, and indecency of language and bearing, of every sort of impropriety—all making up the sum of a career which has become the very antithesis of that of which it is the sequence.

There has been some difference of opinion as to whether this change of habit and character, and these ideational extravagances, do or do not precede the first symptoms of paralysis. I believe that the earliest evidence of disease lies most frequently in the former. It is, of course, I need scarcely tell you, of much importance that you should look out for the primary indication of that impairment of speech which is at once so significant and so fatal. You may fail to see it at your first interview, but observe it at your second; or you may observe it at your first, and not be equally successful at your second; for the manifestation of this symptom varies during its initiatory period with the emotional state of the mind at particular times. But I think I am right in saying that in nearly all cases there is a want of expression about the face, a flatness or tameness of feature, more marked in the upper lip than elsewhere. The patient seems to speak without bringing into play the muscles ordinarily employed in effecting speech. "The eyes have a vacant and absent expression, the pupils being often unequally dilated; the angles of the mouth are sluggish in their movements, the risor and levator anguli oris muscles not appearing to act at all; the mouth opens and shuts in a piece, as it were, without any play of the lips indicative of the sentiments and passions. Not unfrequently the face trembles before speaking, as if the person were about to cry." And very frequently he does cry and sob bitterly. This impairment of articulation simulates the mumbling and indistinct thickness of speech so common in the inebriate. "There is neither stammering nor hesitation of speech," says Dr. Bucknill; "it more closely resembles the thickness of speech observable in a drunken man. It depends upon a loss of power over the co-ordinate action of the muscles of vocal articulation. In many instances the speech of the early paralytic is fluent and clear, except in the pronunciation of certain words, or sequences of words, which require the neat and precise action of the muscles of speech. Words composed of vocal sounds connected by single consonants are articulated with correctness; but words composed of numerous consonants, with few vocalic sounds, are articulated in a shuffling manner, which is perfectly characteristic. The patient may even possess the power of articulating these words correctly, if he purposely attempts to do so; but if the examiner holds him in conversation for a few minutes, the ear will infallibly detect the slight but fatal symptoms of incurable disease. Some little practice in the wards of an asylum is needful to the attainment of readiness in the appreciation of a physical symptom of this kind, just as all the verbal descriptions ever given in books of stethoscopy are of little value, unless the ear is itself practised on the chest of the patient labouring under pulmonary or cardiac disease."

In addition to lesion of speech, there is also in this terrible malady lesion of mobility, which specially manifests itself in want of co-ordinating power over the lower limbs. Occasionally this impairment precedes the impairment of articulation, but more commonly it occurs at a later stage. The patient walks unsteadily, though he tries to walk bravely, keeping his eyes fixed upon the point to which he is bound. He "widens his base of support," and does all he can to steady himself and preserve his centre of gravity. The least touch will throw him off his balance, and demonstrate to all but himself the real defect of locomotion. You will not confound this walk, where the patient puts down his heel with a spurious firmness, with the long and laboured drag of spinal paralysis, where the toes have a tendency to catch against the ground. This lesion of mobility is not an invariable occurrence; I frequently see cases where there is little or no evidence of it. So, likewise, the impairment of articulate speech may scarcely manifest itself, or the grandiose ideas may barely have any existence. With the progressive paralysis, which gradually impairs vocal articulation and locomotion, further evidence is furnished of loss of power. The handwriting sensibly fails—just as words are slurred over and run together in speech, letters and words are dropped in the stenographic performances of the subject of this malady. This failure is clearly a combined defect of perception, and memory, and muscular co-ordination. It is very interesting to compare the writings of these patients from time to time, to notice how the characters gradually cease to maintain their former adjustment and juxtaposition, and how language at last really serves to "conceal thought." Although the early stage of this disease is frequently characterized by moroseness of temper, and violent and ungovernable fits of passion, its second and third stages are not equally obnoxious to these storms and tempests. With increasing grandeur of idea, and the felt presence of boundless wealth, comes increasing calmness and satisfaction. Not the least trying circumstance in connection with general paralysis is the destructiveness which is so persistent and irremediable. It is a common thing to find patients in the morning with their bedding torn to shreds and their mattresses picked in pieces. They will strip themselves, and tie these shreds around various parts of the person, and appear to derive from this fantastic and expensive habit the most lively satisfaction. Even the strong quilted rugs which we substitute for ordinary bedding are not proof against the tearing capacity of the general paralytic. His nights are almost invariably disturbed; he is noisy and clamorous, and destructive of everything within his reach.

The third and closing act of this eventful drama is, as I said before, of less varied incident—the delusions are still present, the grandiose ideas are there, but the power of giving expression to them is lessened, and even the sanguine temperament is dulled and clouded by that fatuity which precedes and heralds the final issue. The powers of articulation and motion are sensibly lessened, the ideas are confused, the perceptive faculties are almost annihilated, and, when spoken to, the patient apprehends only with difficulty what is said to him. There is frequent grinding of the teeth, conveying to the listener a most distressing sensation.

During this later stage (and, indeed, not infrequently during the second) the case becomes complicated with what are termed epileptiform seizures. Dr. Skae, from whose monograph I have before quoted, thus speaks of them :

"These epileptiform or congestive attacks to which general paralytics are liable vary much in frequency and degree in different cases. In some patients they are very frequent, occurring every three or four weeks; in others they are very rare, occurring only once or twice in the whole course of the malady. In some cases they are very slight: the patient complains of pain in the head and confusion of ideas; his face becomes very red and congested; he looks stupid, and perhaps cries without any cause; and after a few hours in bed he recovers his usual composure. In other cases, with more or less congestion of the countenance and confusion of thought, there is a temporary loss of speech, lasting only a few minutes, or passing off after an hour's sleep. In the more completely developed attacks of this affection there is a total loss of consciousness, with convulsive twitchings of the muscles of the face or limbs, varying from one or two slight attacks to repeated and very violent convulsions, lasting for hours, and accompanied with great venous congestion of the scalp and face. These epileptiform attacks are very characteristic, and have been regarded by some writers on the subject as essential features, and diagnostic only of this disease."

It should be mentioned, also, how frequently they are associated with complete hemiplegia. And it is interesting to note how, sometimes in the course of a few hours, after a purgative enema, the completely suspended faculties and locomotive power resume their offices; the hemiplegia disappears, and the patient seems to be little worse for an attack which might have led you to suppose, from the gravity of the symptoms, that a vessel had given way, and deposited a large clot in the cerebral structure. But it is very rarely that anything of this sort is found upon post-mortem examination. The correct explanation of this arrest of power would seem to lie in defect of nutrition. There is probably an interference with the blood-flow in the minute capillaries; the nerve-fibrillæ are thus deprived of their stimulus, and cease to obey the mandates of the will, as also to execute those functions which are independent of the will. When the blood-current is resumed, the nervous executive is gradually resumed likewise—again to break down at varying intervals in the progressive stages of disease. These convulsive seizures have not the same violence as those which are termed epileptic; there is also an absence of the *aura*, and of those jaw movements which produce injury of the tongue. It may here be incidentally mentioned that in the "progressive paralysis" observed in hospitals, an epileptiform seizure is frequently the first external manifestation of the disease.

Gradually, day by day, there is greater helplessness, greater impairment of memory and perception; the stumbling gait, the inarticulate speech, the grinding of the teeth, all attest the downward course of a hopeless malady. The grandiose ideas, the ambitious dreams, may now cease to occupy him; increasing dementia is ejecting, one by one, the former tenants of the disordered mind. A smile may pass over the expressionless face at the mention of them, but it dies away, and all is blank fatuity. It is with difficulty now that the erect position can be maintained; the patient crawls on the floor, makes and remakes the bed on which he never lies, and picks up splinters from the boards. The skin becomes more greasy, and more highly charged with that unmistakable fetor which is so sickening. Nor is the fetor of the breath less distinctive or less disagreeable. Often there is a glutinous secretion round the eyelids, with congestion of the conjunctivæ. Not seldom there is ptosis of one eye, and the vision is defective. The fatty tissues, which so long gave to the patient a characteristic puffiness, are now taken up and appropriated. The appetite continues ravenous, and if not carefully watched and fed, the patient will cram his food into his mouth and choke himself. The reflex action of the muscles concerned in deglutition is less sensitive, and accumulations may take place in the pharynx and produce asphyxia. The actual occurrence of fatal casualties from the impaction of food may be infrequent, but the narrow escapes from these casualties are by no means rare. This tendency to ravenous feeding and the bolting of large masses is very marked in the earlier stages of general paralysis; in the last stage, the food must be chopped very small and soft, almost to liquidness. You will note towards this latter period, as further indicative of general debility, the tendency of the skin to show marks and bruises produced by the very slightest causes. The formation of bullæ containing dark and discoloured serum, of abscesses containing fetid pus, and of ulcers on the leg and elsewhere, is also common. The skin becomes erythematous over the sacrum and great trochanters, and large bedsores ultimately develop themselves. The difficulty of retaining upon them local applications is very great, for the patient is constantly picking them off, and trying to achieve, in a now feeble and less active form, all the mischief of which his helplessness is capable. You must protect these parts from pressure as far as may be by placing him on a water-bed, or, if he has locomotive power, on an air-mattress upon the floor. It is scarcely necessary to state that all power over the bladder and rectum has long been lost; and this circumstance is most unfavourable to the treatment of bedsores. And as he there lies, the veriest wreck that can be conceived of, with his legs doubled, and his knees drawn up against his chin, you will be struck with the position of the head—raised from the pillow, and not resting upon it. Visit the patient when you may, the sterno-cleidomastoids stand out in hard outline, and this elevation may be noted. Sleep seems to have left him, as though it were not needful to anticipate that long and interminable sleep which is so soon to follow.

These are the sad and sickening realities which, unless the patient dies in one of the epileptiform seizures previously spoken of, constitute the closing scene of a drama beginning so ambitiously, and swelling in its rolling course with so much exaltation and pride.

Now, there has been a great difference of opinion as to whether this distressing malady is or is not curable. The late Dr. Sutherland used to say that he had cured cases, and he regarded the bichloride of mercury (perchloride, B.P.) as the agent capable of effecting so satisfactory a result. No one can have a greater respect for the memory of that accomplished physician than I have, for I followed his teaching and saw his practice at St. Luke's Hospital, and he subsequently confided and recommended private patients to my care. But I cannot help thinking that he confounded amelioration with recovery, or that in the cases in which absolute recovery took place there had never really existed the genuine disease with which we are so familiar. For it is beyond a doubt that there is a form of chronic alcoholism in which the earlier symptoms of general paralysis are simulated to a most extraordinary extent. The facial tremor, the thickened speech, the dazed and confused look, the unsteady gait, with hallucinations and delusions—all are there to make up a totality of symptoms which are almost, if not absolutely, identical with the most fatal of diseases. Under care and discipline, and abstinence from the poison which has been so long undermining the citadel of health, aided by fresh air and exercise, and notably the use of the Turkish bath, a great improvement takes place, and, indeed, complete restoration. But of the genuine disease known as general paralysis I agree with Dr. Skae in thinking that the "temporary recoveries are more apparent than real." Certainly I have seen cases where so great a change has resulted from perfect retirement and repose, with the many adjuvants of asylum discipline, that, under the pressing importunity of friends, I have discharged patients *apparently* sound, but in whom the morbific processes have only been for a while suspended. Where friends are so sanguine, and earnest, and loving, one cannot help yielding to them; and there is no reason why such a patient should not again essay the life-battle, and be gifted once more with the pleasant surroundings of family and home.

But the continuity of health is soon broken, or rather the unreality of supposed health is soon made manifest. It is one thing to be fit for home and its social enjoyments, but quite another to be equal to the work of mind and body which may be necessary for the maintenance of a family. There is another circumstance in connection with this sad relapse which must not be lost sight of. I am persuaded that the indulgence of the sexual passion which follows upon a husband's return to his own bed is highly prejudicial to the maintenance of his physical integrity. The attendant exhaustion of nerve-power soon shows itself, and the suppressed symptoms speedily reappear. The case of which I spoke to you just now—of a man who says his legs are golden, that he made the world, &c.—was a striking instance of the deceptive nature of these so-called recoveries from general paralysis of the insane. Certainly I never saw a more remarkable instance of the total disappearance of the gravest symptoms after treatment of six months' duration. When he left the asylum the only perceptible abnormality was unequal dilatation of the pupils. I knew by the loving nature of the young wife what fatal joys were in store for her lord, and hinted to her as delicately as I could of discreetness and moderation. This patient was not brought back to the Asylum for nearly five months; but I gathered that in less than a fortnight from his discharge he was even to his friends manifestly insane.

Some years ago I met out at an evening party a physician whom I knew to have been recently discharged from a lunatic asylum as recovered. I congratulated him upon his return to the outside world, and expressed a hope that he was now quite strong. He laughed at the idea of supposing anything had ever been wrong with him; said he was "first-rate," and so strong that he could lift a sack of flour in each hand. I observed that his pupils were unequally dilated, and I had no doubt whatever that he was then suffering from general paralysis. In ten months' time I observed a notice of his death in the columns of the *Times*.

But there are other authors who say that the genuine disease under consideration is, though very rarely, curable. Buillarger has recorded nine cases; but, in alluding to them, Dr. Sankey says, "It is true that in some of the cases the features of the disease are not strongly marked, but in several at least they were characteristic."

General paralysis of the insane obtains chiefly between the ages of thirty and forty-five. It is rare to meet with it later than sixty or earlier than twenty-five. But cases are on record of its existence under twenty; and I have seen several cases between the age last mentioned and twenty-five. It is much more frequent in men than in women—in the proportion, I think, of at least five to one. Men of the lower class seem to be chiefly obnoxious to it; then we have men of the upper class; thirdly, women of the lower class; whilst, according to Dr. Conolly, the disease is practically unknown amongst women of the highest class. Do fastness and dissoluteness never prevail among the latter? At all events my ladies do not feel the high pressure which exhausts and enervates so many others.

The average duration of general paralysis is about two and a-half years. Some cases, like those of acute phthisis, run their course with marvellous rapidity; others remain stationary for as long as six or seven years. It is said that this malady begins its course as such, and never supervenes upon other forms of insanity. I am not prepared to endorse this statement, though I admit the engrafting, so to speak, of the one disease upon the other is a circumstance of very rare occurrence. Perhaps it might be more accurately put that observers have not detected the fatal symptoms at the earlier period, when they imagined themselves to be dealing with a pathological condition of a more hopeful character. Anyhow, it is certain that many of the subjects of the graver malady have had previous attacks of mania or melancholia, from which they had perfectly recovered.

The causes of general paralysis are varied, and probably made up of a number of combining circumstances, which, as it seems to me, are sufficiently indicated by the fact previously mentioned of the classes most liable to its ravages. Fastness and looseness, wear and tear and high pressure, imperfect nutrition and excessive intemperance and debauch,—what more are wanted to push open the gateway of health and let in disease? Injury to the head and sunstroke are not infrequent causes, but in cases having such an origin the fatuity is developed earlier, and the maniacal symptoms are less acute, and at times altogether absent even in the initiatory stages. Nevertheless I agree with Dr. Blandford in thinking that *per se* sexual excesses have more to do with its causation than anything else.

A wife is indignant if told this, and she appeals to the circumstance that her husband is loyal and faithful. But how does that affect the question at issue? It is not averred that he poaches upon other manors, but simply that he sports too mercilessly and exhaustively upon his own. Uxorious men are given to excesses of a most debilitating nature, and are yet true and faithful. And this is why in cases of apparent improvement, where we have made tentative efforts to restore patients to their homes, there is so frequently a speedy relapse. This exhaustion of nervous energy, then, from a legitimate but too free indulgence of the sexual appetite, together with its illegitimate indulgence by the pernicious habit of self-abuse, are the causal phenomena chiefly concerned in the factorship of this fatal malady. Intemperance, indeed, has much to answer for in the production of insanity, and I have no doubt that the habit is year by year increasing. Consider, with these two powerful agents, the high pressure at which the social wheels are revolving, and you have enough to account for all that we are familiar with under the name of general paralysis of the insane.

As regards the treatment of this disease, being told of its hopelessness, you will see that the agents at our disposal are only palliative. It seems to me that in its earlier stages, during the paroxysms of excitement then so frequent, more good is effected by the tincture of digitalis than anything else. You may disguise its exhibition by putting it in the patient's beer at dinner and supper, where (as so often) he refuses to take it as a separate medicine. In some cases chloral is more useful. The wet sheet is also a very valuable adjuvant in the summer time, during the initiatory period of this malady. The heat of the skin is sometimes abnormally high, there is great excitement, and there is a destructive tendency. In such cases I do not know anything more desirable than to pack these patients after the manner known to hydropathists. The late Dr. Sutherland's great remedy was the bichloride of mercury, but I confess I have not seen the good effects he attributed to it, and I should never think of resorting to such an agent.

One thing above all others is pretty certain respecting these cases, and that is that they are admirably suited to be under asylum discipline and management. The demonstrative nature of the symptoms, and the extravagant nature of the acts of the general paralytic, make him extremely unfit to be at large, even under the surveillance of friends or paid guardians and attendants. He will be far more comfortable in a good asylum, and his relations will be relieved thereby from the occurrence of overt acts and outrageous freaks, which the greatest vigilance outside an asylum cannot always anticipate.

There can be no doubt that the incurable nature of this disease lies in the circumstance that the brain-changes and general deterioration of nerve-element are greater than in any other disease. What most strikes one in examining the brain of a general paralytic is the œdema of the tissues, the enormous amount of serum which escapes upon opening the investing membranes, the patulosity of the cerebral interstices, and the dilatation of the lateral ventricles. The brain in most cases—especially in those where the fatuous period has been protracted—is completely waterlogged. It should be stated the ophthalmoscope reveals optic atrophy as an accompaniment of this disease. It may not be actually demonstrated, but there is good reason to suppose, that the spinal cord and the entire sympathetic system are equally involved with the supreme centres. The vascular changes in the cortical substance of the hemispheres, and the increase of connective tissue in both the grey and white matter, have been dwelt upon by some authors as distinctive of this disease. But it

M

is pretty certain that these changes are not confined to the general paralytic. Dr. Westphal thinks it highly probable that the vaso-motor ganglia are first affected. The pathology, however, of this fatal malady has not yet been clearly defined; and it is more than probable that when (if ever) it is defined, the circumstance will in no way affect its incurability. The ills and the evils of life—excesses, privations, troubles—are the factors of disturbance which lead to the degeneration of normal structure, and constitute what we term disease. We are striving to discover, through the medium of a magnifying power, things and conditions which are rather within the range of social science than the microscope. Much as this little instrument has done for us, I sometimes think we are asking and expecting from it too much, and submitting to its determination problems which can find their solution elsewhere.

LECTURE VII.

Idiocy and Imbecility.

I do not think that in lectures which (as I told you at the outset) are intended to give you a practical and compendious sketch of those mental derangements which are likely to constitute some of the emergencies of general practice, it can be necessary for me to say much to you about idiocy and imbecility. You know to what an extent the training of the most sinless and least responsible of our fellow-creatures has been carried at Earlswood, and other asylums specially devoted to congenital and early deficiencies of brain-structure and power. It will suffice to tell you that idiocy is, strictly speaking, what Esquirol defined it to be— "not a disease, but a condition in which the intellectual faculties are never manifested, or have never been developed sufficiently to enable the idiot to acquire such an amount of knowledge as persons of his own age, and placed in similar circumstances with himself, are capable of receiving."

A sad and piteous spectacle, indeed, are these

blighted waifs, making up a great army of helplessness, appealing through their friends in the columns of the daily papers for means to insure that peculiar education of which some forms of idiocy are susceptible. Formerly some member of this unhappy class was to be met with upon almost every village green, exposed to the jeers and jests of passers-by. But the law has now made provision for them in the different county and borough asylums, as also, more recently, in the metropolitan district, by the erection of institutions for the care and shelter of harmless imbeciles. It is impossible to study the ancestral bearings of these defective creatures without arriving at the conclusion that they are, for the more part, the outcome of a defiance of physiological and sanitary and social laws, and that they furnish the strongest evidence of the truth of the Mosaic declaration—that the sins of the parents are visited upon the generations which succeed them.

Imbecility, as distinguished from idiocy, is not congenital. It is an arrest of functional development, and not an original absence of structure sufficiently sound to execute functions. It is a higher form of organic life, susceptible of more improvement and cultivation. Both of these states are largely associated with epilepsy. This terrible scourge, indeed,—justly termed by Esquirol, in its association with insanity, *le désespoir des médecins*—is a large factor of that arrest of power and subsequent disintegration which eventuate in complete fatuity.

<u>Idiocy</u>, then, is that congenital deficiency which is expressed by the absence of power. <u>Imbecility</u> is the arrest of power before complete development has been attained. <u>Dementia</u> is the final lapse and subversion of power—after a life, it may be, of high intellectual manifestation.

Of the latter condition I have already spoken; and for a study of the two former I must refer you to the recognised text-books. I will just mention, however, that the imbecile class includes a number of persons about whose condition you may have some difficulty in certifying, though you may have no doubt of their mental feebleness and their utter moral depravity. You will be brought into professional contact with them in this way.

A youth of the Wyndham type — known by everyone to be reckless and extravagant, to have no interest in anything but low pursuits and animal enjoyments, and commonly regarded by his friends as "not quite right"—is found to have committed some overt act by which he places himself within the pale of the law; and you are called in your professional capacity to examine him and give evidence as to his state of mind. There are no cases requiring greater judgment and discretion than these; none about which it behoves you to be more careful; none which will expose you to a severer cross-examination in the witness-box. On the one side, it will be urged by friends that the prisoner has always been of feeble capacity, of eager and restless temperament, unable to settle to anything; that he has been untruthful, passionate, addicted to vicious habits, violent antipathies, sundry acts of cruelty and perverseness, and a general obliquity of moral vision, which have often led them to regard his mental condition with much doubt and anxiety. Much colour will be given to the truthfulness of this history by the utterly purposeless and absurd act in which matters have now culminated—such as attempting to intimidate the Queen and obtain her signature to a political document, or upsetting a railway train at full speed, or killing and mutilating an inoffensive child. On the other side, it will be urged that to attempt to set up a plea of insanity in cases of this kind is to offer an apology for crime, and open the door to every sort of outrage. The prisoner has a thorough knowledge of the difference between right and wrong. He knows the value of money, and the amount of enjoyment he can obtain through its means. He has neither delusions, nor illusions, nor hallucinations. The most that can be said is that he has strong impulses to purposeless and vicious acts. You are asked to give an opinion as to whether his volition is so much impaired by disease as to destroy his responsibility and leave him no longer a free agent. And, indeed, you will be asked more than this. It will be put to you more definitely: "Does the prisoner know the difference between right and wrong? Did he know at the time he committed the act with which he was charged that he was doing that which he ought not to have done?" Before you can answer this question, or give any opinion at all upon the case before you, it is of much importance that you should ascertain whether there is any hereditary taint of insanity, or epilepsy, or hysteria, and what are the general health-surroundings of the entire family. You may derive much assistance in determining as to the responsibility of your patient from a complete investigation of these circumstances. But you must remember that the judges and the public are very unwilling to accept the plea of irresponsibility in any cases of insanity—much less in cases where there are no illusions or delusions or hallucinations; and that the law, as laid down by the former, making the knowledge of right and wrong the test of responsibility, is taken exception to by the profession to which you and I belong. Our test is the existence or otherwise of a form of insanity which has impaired the volition, irrespective of the inner consciousness of the difference between good and evil. So strong, indeed, is the feeling against the plea of insanity in criminal cases, that irascible men and women, with small brains and smaller sympathy, are beginning to agitate for uniform punishment, whether madness exists or not. Only a few weeks since I heard at a dinner-table a member of Parliament, while he was sipping his burgundy, maintain this doctrine with an ungenerosity which he could not have derived from his wine. There is reason, however, to think (as I have before had occasion to remark) that this state of feeling has been brought about by an injudicious attempt on the part of alienist physicians to prove too much, and push the plea of insanity beyond its legitimate bounds. All that I can ask you to do in cases of the kind about which I have been speaking, is to look out well and carefully for all the evidences of disease capable of impairing the acts of volition, and, having discovered them, honestly and fearlessly advance them. Responsibility is to be measured by abnormalities of nerve-element, and not by consciousness, for it is certain that (as Dr. Sankey has well expressed it in his lectures) "the most insane act of the insanest individual is nearly always done with a knowledge of whether it is right or wrong." We could not manage asylums as we do if the opinion so commonly entertained by outsiders were true---that mad persons have lost all knowledge of good and evil, and are unamenable to moral control. We must never lose sight of the vast difference between the impairment of a sense or function and its extinction. There is reason to hope that ere long there will be some further legislation upon a subject about which the legal profession is uneasy, the medical profession dissatisfied, and the general public bewildered.

The rules which guide you in determining the criminal responsibility of weak-minded persons will equally serve you in forming a judgment as to their fitness to have the management of property, or their competency for making a testamentary disposition of it.

This will terminate what I have to say on the subject of imbecility.

Criminal Responsibility in Homicidal Mania.

I have already spoken to you, when treating of what is termed moral insanity, of those emotional disturbances, unaccompanied by intellectual derangement, which lead to various impulsive acts, and notably to homicide and self-destruction. And having just now touched upon the overt acts of the weak-minded, occasionally culminating in homicide and suicide likewise, it seems to me that it will be better at once to complete the subject of aggressive violence by again briefly bringing under your notice that form of homicidal mania which is associated with delusions and hallucinations.

To these, more commonly than to any other causal phenomena, are due those personal assaults and manifestations of intense fury which characterize at times the conduct of the insane. If you can once fairly make clear the existence of delusions and hallucinations, the subjects of them will be held to be of unsound mind, inasmuch as their presence was formerly held to be the legal test of insanity.

This of itself should be sufficient to establish criminal irresponsibility. But you have observed, I have no doubt, the importation by the judges into these cases of a matter which is really quite foreign to the issue. They enquire of a medical witness, not whether the prisoner is of unsound mind, but whether he is in a position to know the difference between right and wrong. Dr. Blandford has well remarked, "No more curious test of insanity was ever invented—none which more plainly shows the absolute ignorance of the subject prevailing amongst those who have no acquaintance with the insane."

But, happily, the judges are not unanimous in this monstrous view of responsibility, with a blood-stained medico-legal literature, such as we can point to, of crime manifestly resulting from disease; for one of them has, more wisely and humanely than his colleagues, affirmed "that it was not merely for the jury to consider whether the prisoner knew right from wrong, but whether he was at the time he committed the offence deranged or not."

I have told you before that there are really very few lunatics who have not a knowledge, however imperfect, of the difference between right and wrong. When delusions and hallucinations exist to such an extent as to dominate the will and lead to those irresistible "external utterances" which involve the gravest crimes, you will frequently hear the subjects of them acknowledging the wickedness of the deed which they contemplated, and their powerlessness to resist its execution. On the other hand, at times they cannot be convinced of their error, because (as Esquirol remarks) they are persuaded that <u>what they perceive</u> is the legitimate effect of an impression, and that what they would do is just and reasonable. I had a patient the other day who was bent upon killing his wife, *because he had been ordered to do so.* If God (he said) told him to kill her, it *must* be right to do so, and nothing should prevent his doing it. In about two months this aural hallucination disappeared, and his wife was again to him all the world. It was interesting to note in this case (what is so commonly observed in homicidal mania) that the mind was *apparently* sound upon all other subjects, but the one great and racking conviction that wife-slaughter was an heroic act, to be carried out in obedience to a divine command. I say *apparently*, because (as I have before pointed out to you) there must really be various morbid associations and impressions of which a homicidal appetite is the only outcome. It is hardly possible to believe that there is not some lesion both of the intelligence and the affective nature when the culminating desire of this grave derangement is to take away the life of the nearest and dearest. Yet these cases have been described as *mono*maniacal, in allusion to that *desordre dans les actions* (as Esquirol expresses it) to which authors have given the name of *folie raisonnante*, and which so dominates the will by the singleness of its oppression as to exclude all other ideas and considerations.

Feigned Insanity.

You will sometimes, perhaps, be called upon to give your opinion in a case of suspected malingering. To escape punishment, or free himself from a civil obligation, or even from less pressing reasons than these, a man will attempt to feign insanity. Commonly he does not know how difficult and sustained a part he has to play for even a remote chance of success, and the curtain falls upon a grotesque and blundering farce more quickly than he anticipated. Hamlets are not to be met with every day, and our friend has proved unequal to the task which he set himself to do. Those who are acquainted with the genuine article will soon discover how miserably he is overacting his part, tear off the mask, and expose the imposture. Let me beg of you to study these cases carefully, and bring to bear upon them all your discernment and acumen. Bear in mind that cultivated and refined malingerers, such as Shakespeare has depicted the Danish prince, are of very rare occurrence. Our field of observation lies with a very different class —the criminal population; and so intimately leagued are crime and insanity, that many of the worst characters afloat on the surface of the social waters are compounded of a maximum of vice and a minimum of madness.

In a very interesting and instructive article upon the "Hereditary Nature of Crime,"* by Mr. J. B. Thomson, Resident Surgeon to the General Prison for Scotland, at Perth, it is demonstrated that the principal business of prison surgeons lies with mental diseases; that the number of physical diseases is less than the psychical; that the diseases and causes of death among prisoners are chiefly of the nervous system; and, in fine, that *the treatment of crime is a branch of psychology.* I draw your attention to this league between insanity and crime in order that you may be fully prepared to estimate its importance when you are called in by prison surgeons to assist them in coming to a conclusion in a case of suspected malingering. For it is certain that criminals who have a slight taint of alienation, whether hereditary or otherwise, are cunning enough to know the advantage which they may derive from its exaggeration, just as the certified insane will frequently, from very love of spite and mischief, commit assaults upon their attendants, because they know the powerlessness (under pains and penalties) of the latter to retaliate. I have frequently heard one crafty lunatic of the criminal type urge another to aggressive acts upon an attendant, saying, "Pitch into him; he dare not hit you again, because you are a lunatic."

Sometimes, also, you will find persons, who have

* Journal of Mental Science, January, 1870.

committed an offence involving penal consequences, not pretending to be other than perfectly sane at the time you see them, but affirming, with an assumed bewilderment as to what has taken place, that they suppose they must have had some transitory period of unconsciousness, during which they have been guilty of a breach of the law. It has occurred to these artful gentlemen that by pretending an utter ignorance of the crime charged, and an oblivion of recent events, they will be able to evade the punishment to which they are most legitimately entitled. In cases of this sort you must endeavour to ascertain the history of the prisoner, and institute particular inquiries as to whether he has ever been the subject of epilepsy, or any form of convulsive seizure. It is obvious that you cannot get much from the prisoner himself without furnishing him weapons which he will be acute enough to turn to his own advantage.

A more common form of malingering is that in which the prisoner feigns at the time of your visit, with a view to making you believe that his immediate condition is but a continuation of that under which he committed the offence laid to his charge. But he has no intention of keeping up false appearances longer than a few days, when in the natural course of things he will recover, as he knows the really insane do, from a transitory attack of mania or melancholia.

But the malingerers who will give you most

trouble are those scoundrels who know half the prisons in the country, and even many of the asylums, where they have managed for a while to find a comfortable home, and at the same time made a study of insanity with a view of turning it to a profitable account. The courage and perseverance of these fellows under what would seem to be almost overwhelming difficulties is incredible, and only commensurate with their villainy. I have had not a few specimens of this class during my tenure of office in Colney Hatch Asylum.

One of the most remarkable instances on record of persevering simulation is narrated by Dr. Bucknill,* in which he and other medical men were for a time deceived; it is so instructive that I shall place it before you: "W. Warren was a notorious thief, indicted at the Devonshire assizes, 18—, for felony; previous convictions having been proved against him, he was sentenced to transportation for fourteen years. Two days after his trial he all at once became apparently insane; he constantly made howling noises, was filthy in his habits, and destroyed his bedding and clothing; he was, however, suspected of malingering, and was detained in gaol three months. During a part of this time it was found needful to keep him in a strait-waistcoat. At length certificates of his insanity were forwarded to the Secretary of State, and he was ordered to be

* Manual of Pyschological Medicine, by Drs. Bucknill and Tuke, p. 340.

removed to the Devon County Asylum. On admission into this asylum he certainly was very feeble, and in weak health. He had an oppressed and stupid expression of face; he answered no questions, but muttered constantly to himself; he retained the same position for hours, either in a standing or sitting posture; he was not dirty in his habits; he appeared to be suffering from acute dementia. In three weeks' time he recovered bodily strength, and his mind became gradually clear. This change was too rapid not to suggest the idea of deception, but the previous symptoms of dementia had been so true to nature that we still thought the insanity might not have been feigned. For a period of eight months he was well-conducted and industrious, and showed no symptoms of insanity. At the end of that time he was returned to the gaol, to undergo his sentence; and about one hour after readmission within its portals he was apparently affected with a relapse of his mental disease. He refused to answer all questions; walking to and fro in his cell, he constantly muttered to himself, and sometimes made howling noises which disturbed the quiet of the prison. Sometimes he refused his food for days together. He employed his time walking to and fro in his cell, muttering unintelligibly; or in beating at the door of his cell; or in turning his bedclothes over and over, as if looking for something. He had a very stupid expression of face, heightened by inflammation of the eyes, from the lashes growing inwards. He slept soundly. For some months he was very filthy; this habit was cured by the governor of the prison ordering him to be put into a hot bath—hot enough to be painful, but not to scald; he jumped out of the bath with more energy than he had before shown, and thenceforth did not repeat his filthy practices. We visited him several times in prison, and expressed our positive opinion that his insanity was feigned. With the exception of uncleanly habits, he maintained all the symptoms of insanity which he had adopted for two whole years; his resolution then suddenly gave way, he acknowledged his deception, and requested the governor of the prison to forward him as soon as might be to the Government depôt for convicts. In this remarkable case, the perseverance of the simulator, his refusal to converse or to answer questions, and the general truthfulness of his representation, made it most difficult to arrive at a decisive opinion. Still, the rapidity of his recovery, in the first instance, and the suddenness of his relapse, in the second, were inconsistent with the course of that form of insanity to which he presented so striking a resemblance. Our opinion, therefore, was formed upon a history of the case, and not upon any obvious inconsistency in the symptoms."

The cunning and wickedness of some of these malingering adepts (as seen in the above case) is very remarkable. I had a man of this stamp under my care who had been at various asylums and prisons, and prided himself on baffling the doctors and the governors. He had certainly an insane taint, but it was swamped by his villainy. I brought him before the magistrates for discharge. He refused to leave the asylum, and I was under the necessity of having him carried down to the station. There was a nice little game with him on the platform and in the train; and when he got to King's Cross the attendants in whose charge I was sending him to the workhouse placed him in a cab, of which he immediately smashed all the windows. The cabman at once drove him to a police-court, and brought him before the magistrate, who, hearing whence he came, advised his being taken back again, as he was certainly mad; but my officers explained to the magistrate the nature of the case and the rascality of the subject, when, in default of payment, he was committed to prison. I have never heard of the fellow since. He had a long history of eccentric and outrageous crime behind him.

Confessedly, then, even to an experienced alienist physician, the detection of feigned insanity, when cleverly simulated by an adept, may be a matter of much difficulty. But the adepts are few, and the bunglers are many. The part is generally overacted, and is too demonstrative in its manner and bearing. There is a want of coherence and consistency and "method" about it—a clumsy and *bizarre* grouping of symptoms which are not characteristic of one form of insanity only. And there may be some reason for this. It is hard work to play the part of a wild and frenzied maniac for any length of time. A few days of melancholia or dementia are a real and welcome rest to the simulator. It behoves you, in a case of this kind, to carefully examine those who have been about the prisoner, and who have silently watched him. Ascertain if he has slept well; for this matter of sleep is of great diagnostic value. The really maniacal do *not* sleep; the histrionically maniacal *do*. In personating demonstrative disease you lay the faculties under contribution, and those faculties need, and will have, repose. But the genuine disease is the result of disordered faculties, whose first evidence of derangement is the impossibility of repose. What is the state of the skin and the pulse? Did the attack whose reality you are called upon to decide come on suddenly without previous symptoms? Is there any object in simulation—to escape punishment, or get into comfortable quarters in a lunatic asylum? All these matters must be considered before you can really determine whether the conduct of the prisoner before you is the result of disease or wickedness.

While malingerers, then, are met with both in prisons and asylums, it must not, on the other hand, be overlooked that, in the former, persons (notably imbecile youths of low type and imperfect development) are discovered to be undergoing punishment for crimes committed under the absence of moral responsibility. Crime is as hereditary as disease, and is so intimately leagued with it that we do not make sufficient allowance for that "tyranny of a bad organization" which drives its subjects so remorselessly into the ways which are not of pleasantness, and the paths which are not of peace. Few can estimate the struggle which it is, to some feeble natures weighted with the desperate heritage of disease, to keep in a straight line, and preserve a moral equilibrium; while to others, by reason of their somatic integrity, it is comparatively easy to walk steadily and uprightly.

> "How easy 'tis, when destiny proves kind,
> With full-spread sails to run before the wind!"

Not long since I received into Colney Hatch Asylum from one of the prisons an imbecile youth who had there been found incorrigible. Birch and gruel were powerless to effect an improvement, but they rather augmented those vices which were sapping and undermining the little intelligence with which Nature had ever gifted him. Under good diet, and a measure of moral discipline suited to his capacity, he has improved. But you have only to regard his physical conformation, and see that intellectually he is far below the average of a tutored monkey or an educated French poodle. Shapen in iniquity and conceived in sin — the blended product, it may be, of intemperance, and syphilis, and epilepsy,—he is absolutely powerless to rise.

While it will be your duty, then, to detect the malingerers and bring them to justice, you must not lose sight of those who have been deprived of moral responsibility by disease, but do your utmost to bring them within the merciful provisions of the laws of lunacy.

Before bringing these lectures to a conclusion, I am desirous of reverting to the subject of "non-restraint" in the care and treatment of the insane; for I happen to be one of those who—as humane, I trust, as other alienist physicians—think that much evil has resulted from its too rigid adoption. I am almost prepared to endorse the statement made to me in his own asylum—one of the best conducted in Germany—by its physician and medical superintendent: "You have a monomania in England, my dear doctor, and it is called 'non-restraint.'"

It was, indeed, the custom formerly to restrain lunatics in a most reckless and indiscriminate manner, in order to save trouble. They were neglected because they were restrained; but in the exceptional cases of restraint now practised they are restrained in order that they may not be neglected. For it *is* to neglect them if we fail in adopting those measures which best meet the requirements of safety and decency. It is a perver sion of terms to call any system humane which does not do this. And in order to estimate the value of such a system, we have to inquire what other means are at our disposal for certain aggravated forms of homicidal mania, or suicidal melancholia, or persistent destructiveness. They are two—both at times tremendously and dangerously coercive—both entitled to be regarded as "restraints" in the truest sense of the term, but involving no official entry in the "medical journal." Hence the preference so naturally and so commonly given to them. 1st, There is the "chemical restraint," resulting from large and repeated doses of sedatives and narcotics, which so frequently "make havoc among those tender cells" of which the human brain is compounded. 2nd. There is the uncertain supervision of one or more special attendants, who may drop asleep, or lose their temper, and by unnecessary officiousness provoke frequent struggles with their charge. Many of the broken ribs and other casualties in English asylums, which have given rise to so much comment and censure, moving the facile pens of novelists, and stimulating the imaginations of their readers, have resulted from struggles between attendants and patients, which would have been avoided, and ought to have been avoided, by temporary mechanical restraint. I have had suicidal patients implore me to restrain them, under impulses which they desired but were powerless to control. The persistent aggressiveness of a dangerous epileptic lately under my charge has necessitated "instrumental coercion" to a very exceptional extent. Such a method was not resorted to till all other methods had failed, and has been attended by the most satisfactory results, although it has provoked the official comments of the Commissioners in Lunacy.

There is not the least doubt in my own mind that as "blood-letting," until recently, has been too absolutely abolished under all pathological conditions for more than a quarter of a century, so the "non-restraint" system has been too closely adhered to under all emergencies. History even here does but repeat itself, by showing that the surrender of one extreme invariably leads to the adoption of another. The two extremes have been tried: a healthier reaction is bringing us to the rational mean. Blood-letting is now recognised as sometimes useful; "restraint" is acknowledged by all of large experience to be, under certain conditions, both salutary and humane. In cases of persistent suicidal and homicidal impulses, valuable lives are frequently preserved by the temporary adoption of what is termed "instrumental coercion." That treatment, I repeat, cannot in the largest sense be called humane which does not make the most effective provision against these aggressive outbreaks. It is wiser to be cautious against surprises than to be afterwards surprised into caution. One of the Commissioners recently told me of a case where their advice that a determined suicide should be subjected to mechanical restraint had been neglected at the cost of life. And I tell you—what a large experience justifies me in telling you—that you will be highly culpable if, through fear of official censure, you neglect to resort to this means of treatment when your judgment tells you that it is necessary. We shall never improve if we are not honest enough and bold enough to promulgate and sustain our true convictions.*

There are several matters in connection with the insane, their management, and the general administration of places devoted to their care and wellbeing, which it may be instructive for me in the last place to touch upon. For you should know that

---

* An experienced medical superintendent of one of our largest asylums (Dr. Rogers, Rainhill, Lancashire) has recently written:—"The liability to *abuse* of any agent or system forms no adequate ground for its rejection, if its *use* can be proved to be really beneficial; and if a man has satisfied himself on sufficient evidence that restraint or seclusion, blood-letting or alcohol, narcotics, purgatives, tonics, or any other mode of treatment is beneficial to his patients, I hold that he ought to act according to his own judgment, without regard to the *fashion* of treatment prevailing in his days." Dr. Yellowlees, of the Glamorgan County Asylum, Dr. Lindsay, of the Derby County Asylum, and many other superintendents, have written to the same effect. The resident physicians of the American asylums are likewise convinced (to quote one of them—Dr. Chapin, King's County) that mechanical restraint is sometimes most salutary, and that experience has proved beyond a doubt that "it can only be dispensed with to a greater extent than was before deemed possible." "What I saw in Europe," continues Dr. Chapin, "tended to strengthen my previous conviction that instances do occasionally everywhere occur in which the best interests of insane persons require the use of mechanical restraints."

lunatics *do* require singular care and management; and it is beyond a doubt that a man may have a first-rate knowledge of his profession, be a ripe scholar and able physician, and yet be very unsuited to have charge of an asylum, or to have any dealings with the insane. You must remember that, for the more part, deranged persons, not being melancholic or demented, have all their faculties highly acute and sensitive. They are keenly observant, and are on the look out for every weakness and blunder on your part, which they will not fail to turn to your disadvantage.

An alienist physician should be a physiognomist and a great observer of character. Men and manners should be his specialty. He should know when and how to say the right thing, bearing in mind that words which are suited to one may be eminently unsuited to another. It is wonderful what influence and real hold upon a patient may be obtained by a happy remark, or a judicious shrug of the shoulders, or a kind and sympathizing look, or a reserved and dignified bearing—according to their respective needs for respective cases. I remember once giving mortal offence to a morbid religionist of the old Puritan type by an injudicious remark upon the school to which he belonged. He never forgave me, and took such a rooted dislike to me that I was under the necessity of requesting the magistrates to transfer him to the sister asylum at Hanwell.

Nor are less tact and judgment required in managing the staff of attendants under whose charge you have to place your patients. They give at times an infinity of trouble, and are guilty of indiscretions and improprieties which are anything but creditable to their common sense or humanity. But you must bear in mind that they are placed not infrequently in most trying positions, and are liable to have charges made against them which have little or no foundation in truth. These charges must be investigated with the greatest caution and strictness, and, as a rule, it will be dangerous and unjust ever to accept the unsupported testimony of a lunatic. Epileptic religionists are never to be relied upon, for they are the most untruthful, as the most afflicted, of human beings.

And so I bring these lectures to a close. It is not pretended that they have done more, or can ever do more, than give you a general outline of those maladies which go to make up what is termed "insanity." For more detailed information you must consult the recognised text-books. The subject itself has, I trust, enlisted your sympathies and your interest. The more you study it, the more it will recommend itself to you; for there is nothing nobler to which you can devote your faculties than the ministering to minds which are afflicted with disease.

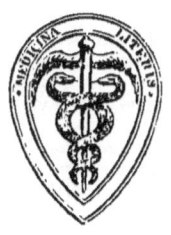

London, New Burlington Street.
September, 1879.

SELECTION

FROM

MESSRS J. & A. CHURCHILL'S

General Catalogue

COMPRISING

ALL RECENT WORKS PUBLISHED BY THEM

ON THE

ART AND SCIENCE

OF

MEDICINE

INDEX

	PAGE
Acton on the Reproductive Organs	8
Adams (W.) on Clubfoot	6
— (R.) on Rheumatic Gout	19
Allingham on Diseases of the Rectum	7
Anatomical Remembrancer	11
Anderson (McC.) on Eczema	20
Aveling's Influence of Posture	15
Balfour's Diseases of the Heart	17
Bantock's Rupture of Perineum	14
Barclay's Medical Diagnosis	12
Barker's Puerperal Diseases	13
Barnes' Obstetric Operations	14
— Diseases of Women	14
Basham on Diseases of the Kidneys	8
Beale's Microscope in Medicine	11
Bellamy's Guide to Surgical Anatomy	10
Bennet's Winter and Spring on the Mediterranean	17
— Pulmonary Consumption	17
— Nutrition	18
Berkart's Asthma	16
Bigg's Orthopraxy	6
Binz's Elements of Therapeutics	12
Black on the Urinary Organs	8
Blakiston's Clinical Reminiscences	11
Bose's Rational Therapeutics	11
— Recognisant Medicine	11
Bradley's Lymphatic System	15
Braune's Topographical Anatomy	11
Brodhurst's Orthopædic Surgery	6
Bryant's Practice of Surgery	4
Bucknill and Tuke's Psychological Medicine	21
Burdett's Cottage Hospital	15
Burnett on the Ear	6
Buzzard on Syphilitic Nervous Affections	8
Carpenter's Human Physiology	10
Carter (W.) on Renal and Urinary Diseases	8
Charteris' Practice of Medicine	11
Clark's Outlines of Surgery	4
— Surgical Diagnosis	5
Clay's Obstetric Surgery	13
Cobbold on Parasites	20
Coles' Dental Mechanics	23
Cormack's Clinical Studies	12
Cullingworth's Nurse's Companion	15
Curling's Diseases of the Rectum	7
— Diseases of the Testis	7
Dalby on the Ear	6
Dalton's Human Physiology	9
Day on Children's Diseases	13
— on Headaches	18
Dobell's Lectures on Winter Cough	15
— Loss of Weight, &c.	15
Domville's Manual for Hospital Nurses	15
Druitt's Surgeon's Vade-Mecum	4
Duncan on the Female Perineum	15
Dunglison's Medical Dictionary	22
Ellis's Manual of Diseases of Children	13
Emmet's Gynæcology	14
Eulenburg and Guttmann's Sympathetic System of Nerves	19
Fayrer's Observations in India	4
Fergusson's Practical Surgery	4
Fenwick's Guide to Medical Diagnosis	12
Flint on Phthisis	16
— on Percussion and Auscultation	16
Foster's Clinical Medicine	11
Fox (C. B.) Sanitary Examinations	21
Fox (T.) Atlas of Skin Diseases	20
Fox (T.) and Farquhar's Skin Diseases of India	20
Frey's Histology	9
Galabin's Diseases of Women	14
Gamgee on Fractures of the Limbs	4
— on Treatment of Wounds	4
Gant's Diseases of the Bladder	8
Gaskoin on Psoriasis or Lepra	20
Godlee's Atlas of Human Anatomy	11
Gowan on Consumption	16
Gowers' Medical Ophthalmoscopy	21
Habershon on Diseases of the Abdomen	18
— on Diseases of the Stomach	18
— on the Pneumogastric Nerve	18
Hamilton's Nervous Diseases	18
Hancock's Surgery of Foot and Ankle	6
Harris on Lithotomy	7
Harrison's Stricture of Urethra	7
Hayden on the Heart	16
Heath's Minor Surgery and Bandaging	5
— Diseases and Injuries of Jaws	5
— Operative Surgery	5
— Surgical Diagnosis	5
— Practical Anatomy	10
Higgens' Ophthalmic Practice	22
Holden's Landmarks	10
— Human Osteology	10
Hood on Gout, Rheumatism, &c.	19
Hooper's Physician's Vade-Mecum	11
Horton's Tropical Diseases	18
Hutchinson's Clinical Surgery	5
— Rare Diseases of Skin	20
Huth's Marriage of Near Kin	8
Ireland's Idiocy and Imbecility	20
James' Sore Throat	17
Jones (C. H.) and Sieveking's Pathological Anatomy	10
Jones (H. McN.) Aural Surgery	6
— Atlas of Diseases of Membrana Tympani	6
Jordan's Surgical Inquiries	6
Lane on Syphilis	8
Leber and Rottenstein's Dental Caries	23
Lee (H.) on Syphilis	8
Leared on Imperfect Digestion	19

	PAGE
Liveing on Megrim, &c.	19
Macdonald's (A.) Disease of the heart	16
Macdonald's (J. D.) Examination of Water	21
Mackenzie on Diphtheria	16
Macnamara on Diseases of the Eye	22
Madden's Health Resorts	17
Marsden on certain Forms of Cancer	19
Mason on Harelip and Cleft Palate	5
— Surgery of the Face	5
Maunder's Operative Surgery	4
— Surgery of Arteries	4
Mayne's Medical Vocabulary	22
Morris (H.) Anatomy of the Joints	10
Ogston's Medical Jurisprudence	20
Osborn on Hydrocele	7
Parkes' Manual of Practical Hygiene	21
Pavy on Food and Dietetics	19
— on Diabetes	19
Peacock's Valvular Disease	16
Pirrie's Surgery	4
Pollock's Rheumatism	19
Ramsbotham's Obstetrics	13
Reynolds' Uses of Electricity	22
Roberts' (C.) Manual of Anthropometry	9
Roberts' (D. Lloyd) Practice of Midwifery	13
Roussel's Transfusion of Blood	5
Routh's Infant Feeding	13
Royle and Harley's Materia Medica	12
Rutherford's Practical Histology	9
Salt's Medico-Electric Apparatus	22
Sanderson's Physiological Handbook	9
Sansom's Diseases of the Heart	17
Savage on the Female Pelvic Organs	4
Savory's Domestic Medicine	15
Sayre's Orthopædic Surgery	6
Schroeder's Manual of Midwifery	13
Semple on the Heart	16
Sewill's Dental Anatomy	23
Shapter's Diseases of the Heart	16
Sheppard on Madness	21
Sibson's Medical Anatomy	10
Sieveking's Life Assurance	21
Smith (E.) Wasting Diseases of Children	13
— Clinical Studies	13
Smith (Henry) Surgery of the Rectum	8
Smith (Heywood) Gynæcology	14
Smith (J.) Dental Anatomy	23
Smith (W. R.) Nursing	15
Spender's Bath Waters	17
Steiner's Diseases of Children	13
Stillé and Maisch's National Dispensatory	12

	PAGE
Stocken's Dental Materia Medica	12
Sullivan's Tropical Diseases	17
Swain's Surgical Emergencies	5
Swayne's Obstetric Aphorisms	14
Taft's Operative Dentistry	23
Tait's Hospital Mortality	15
Taylor's Principles of Medical Jurisprudence	20
— Manual of Medical Jurisprudence	20
— Poisons in relation to Medical Jurisprudence	20
Teale's Dangers to Health	21
Thomas on Ear and Throat Diseases	6
Thompson's Practical Lithotomy and Lithotrity	7
— Diseases of Urinary Organs	7
— Diseases of the Prostate	7
— Calculous Disease	7
Thornton on Tracheotomy	17
Thorowgood on Asthma	16
— on Materia Medica	12
Thudichum's Pathology of Urine	8
Tibbits' Medical Electricity	22
— Map of Motor Points	22
Tilt's Uterine Therapeutics	14
— Change of Life	14
— Health in India	18
Tomes' (C. S.) Dental Anatomy	23
— (J. and C. S.) Dental Surgery	23
Tunstall's Bath Waters	17
Van Buren on Diseases of the Genito-Urinary Organs	8
Veitch's Handbook for Nurses	15
Virchow's Post-mortem Examinations	10
Wagstaffe's Human Osteology	9
Walker's Ophthalmology	23
Walton's Diseases of the Eye	22
Ward on Affections of the Liver	18
Waring's Practical Therapeutics	12
— Bazaar Medicines of India	18
Wells (Soelberg) on Diseases of the Eye	23
— Long, Short, and Weak Sight	23
Wells (Spencer) on Diseases of the Ovaries	14
West and Duncan's Diseases of Women	14
Whistler's Syphilis of the Larynx	17
Wilks' Diseases of Nervous System	18
— Pathological Anatomy	10
Wilson's (E.) Anatomist's Vade-Mecum	11
— Lectures on Dermatology	20
Wilson's (G.) Handbook of Hygiene	22
Woodman & Tidy's Forensic Medicine	21

THE PRACTICE OF SURGERY :
a Manual by THOMAS BRYANT, F.R.C.S., Surgeon to Guy's Hospital. Third Edition, 2 vols., crown 8vo, with 672 Engravings, 28s. [1878]

THE PRINCIPLES AND PRACTICE OF SURGERY,
by WILLIAM PIRRIE, F.R.S.E., Professor of Surgery in the University of Aberdeen. Third Edition, 8vo, with 490 Engravings, 28s. [1873]

A SYSTEM OF PRACTICAL SURGERY,
by Sir WILLIAM FERGUSSON, Bart., F.R.C.S., F.R.S. Fifth Edition, 8vo, with 463 Engravings, 21s. [1870]

OPERATIVE SURGERY,
by C. F. MAUNDER, F.R.C.S., Surgeon to the London Hospital. Second Edition, post 8vo, with 164 Engravings, 6s. [1872]

BY THE SAME AUTHOR.

SURGERY OF THE ARTERIES:
Lettsomian Lectures for 1875, on Aneurisms, Wounds, Hæmorrhages, &c. Post 8vo, with 18 Engravings, 5s. [1875]

THE SURGEON'S VADE-MECUM,
a Manual of Modern Surgery, by ROBERT DRUITT. Eleventh Edition, fcap. 8vo, with 369 Engravings, 14s. [1878]

OUTLINES OF SURGERY AND SURGICAL PATHOLOGY,
including the Diagnosis and Treatment of Obscure and Urgent Cases, and the Surgical Anatomy of some Important Structures and Regions, by F. LE GROS CLARK, F.R.S., Consulting Surgeon to St. Thomas's Hospital. Second Edition, Revised and Expanded by the Author, assisted by W. W. WAGSTAFFE, F.R.C.S., Assistant-Surgeon to St. Thomas's Hospital. 8vo, 10s. 6d. [1872]

CLINICAL AND PATHOLOGICAL OBSERVATIONS IN INDIA,
by Sir J. FAYRER, K.C.S.I., M.D., F.R.C.P. Lond., F.R.S.E., Honorary Physician to the Queen. 8vo, with Engravings, 20s. [1873]

TREATMENT OF WOUNDS:
Clinical Lectures, by SAMPSON GAMGEE, F.R.S.E., Surgeon to the Queen's Hospital, Birmingham. Crown 8vo, with Engravings, 5s. [1878]

BY THE SAME AUTHOR,

FRACTURES OF THE LIMBS
and their Treatment. 8vo, with Plates, 10s. 6d. [1871]

THE FEMALE PELVIC ORGANS,
their Surgery, Surgical Pathology, and Surgical Anatomy, in a Series of Coloured Plates taken from Nature: with Commentaries, Notes, and Cases, by HENRY SAVAGE, M.D. Lond., F.R.C.S., Consulting Officer of the Samaritan Free Hospital. Third Edition, 4to, £1 15s.
[1876]

SURGICAL EMERGENCIES
together with the Emergencies attendant on Parturition and the Treatment of Poisoning: a Manual for the use of General Practitioners, by WILLIAM P. SWAIN, F.R.C.S., Surgeon to the Royal Albert Hospital, Devonport. Second Edition, post 8vo, with 104 Engravings, 6s. 6d. [1876]

TRANSFUSION OF HUMAN BLOOD:
with Table of 50 cases, by Dr. ROUSSEL, of Geneva. Translated by CLAUDE GUINNESS, B.A. With a Preface by SIR JAMES PAGET, Bart. Crown 8vo, 2s. 6d. [1877]

ILLUSTRATIONS OF CLINICAL SURGERY,
consisting of Coloured Plates, Photographs, Woodcuts, Diagrams, &c., illustrating Surgical Diseases, Symptoms and Accidents; also Operations and other methods of Treatment. By JONATHAN HUTCHINSON, F.R.C.S., Senior Surgeon to the London Hospital. In Quarterly Fasciculi, 6s. 6d. each. Fasciculi I to X bound, with Appendix and Index, £3 10s. [1876-9]

PRINCIPLES OF SURGICAL DIAGNOSIS
especially in Relation to Shock and Visceral Lesions, by F. LE GROS CLARK, F.R.C.S., Consulting Surgeon to St. Thomas's Hospital. 8vo, 10s. 6d. [1870]

MINOR SURGERY AND BANDAGING:
a Manual for the Use of House-Surgeons, Dressers, and Junior Practitioners, by CHRISTOPHER HEATH, F.R.C.S., Surgeon to University College Hospital, and Holme Professor of Surgery in University College. Fifth Edition, fcap 8vo, with 86 Engravings, 5s. 6d. [1875]

BY THE SAME AUTHOR,
INJURIES AND DISEASES OF THE JAWS:
JACKSONIAN PRIZE ESSAY. Second Edition, 8vo, with 164 Engravings, 12s. [1872]

BY THE SAME AUTHOR,
A COURSE OF OPERATIVE SURGERY:
with 20 Plates drawn from Nature by M. LÉVEILLÉ, and coloured by hand under his direction. Large 8vo. 40s. [1877]

BY THE SAME AUTHOR,
THE STUDENT'S GUIDE TO SURGICAL DIAGNOSIS.
Fcap. 8vo, 6s. 6d. [1879]

HARE-LIP AND CLEFT PALATE,
by FRANCIS MASON, F.R.C.S., Surgeon and Lecturer on Anatomy at St. Thomas's Hospital. With 66 Engravings, 8vo, 6s. [1877]

BY THE SAME AUTHOR,
THE SURGERY OF THE FACE:
with 100 Engravings. 8vo, 7s. 6d. [1878]

DISEASES AND INJURIES OF THE EAR,
by W. B. DALBY, F.R.C.S., M.B., Aural Surgeon and Lecturer on Aural Surgery at St. George's Hospital. Crown 8vo, with 21 Engravings, 6s. 6d. [1873]

AURAL SURGERY;
A Practical Treatise, by H. MACNAUGHTON JONES, M.D., Professor of the Queen's University in Ireland, Surgeon to the Cork Ophthalmic and Aural Hospital. With 46 Engravings, crown 8vo, 5s. [1878]

BY THE SAME AUTHOR,
ATLAS OF DISEASES OF THE MEMBRANA TYMPANI.
In Coloured Plates, containing 62 Figures, with Text, crown 4to, 21s. [1878]

THE EAR:
its Anatomy, Physiology, and Diseases. A Practical Treatise, by CHARLES H. BURNETT, A.M., M.D., Aural Surgeon to the Presbyterian Hospital, and Surgeon in Charge of the Infirmary for Diseases of the Ear, Philadelphia. With 87 Engravings, 8vo, 18s. [1877]

EAR AND THROAT DISEASES.
Essays by LLEWELLYN THOMAS, M.D., Surgeon to the Central London Throat and Ear Hospital. Post 8vo, 2s. 6d. [1878]

CLUBFOOT ·
its Causes, Pathology, and Treatment: Jacksonian Prize Essay by WM. ADAMS, F.R.C.S., Surgeon to the Great Northern Hospital. Second Edition, 8vo, with 106 Engravings and 6 Lithographic Plates, 15s. [1873]

ORTHOPÆDIC SURGERY:
Lectures delivered at St. George's Hospital, by BERNARD E. BRODHURST, F.R.C.S., Surgeon to the Royal Orthopædic Hospital. Second Edition, 8vo, with Engravings, 12s. 6d. [1876]

OPERATIVE SURGERY OF THE FOOT AND ANKLE,
by HENRY HANCOCK, F.R.C.S., Consulting Surgeon to Charing Cross Hospital. 8vo, with Engravings, 15s. [1873]

SURGICAL INQUIRIES.
By FURNEAUX JORDAN, F.R.C.S., Professor of Surgery in Queen's College, Birmingham. With numerous Lithographic Plates. 8vo, 5s. [1873]

ORTHOPRAXY:
the Mechanical Treatment of Deformities, Debilities, and Deficiencies of the Human Frame, by H. HEATHER BIGG, Associate of the Institute of Civil Engineers. Third Edition, with 319 Engravings, 8vo, 15s. [1877]

ORTHOPÆDIC SURGERY ·
and Diseases of the Joints. Lectures by LEWIS A. SAYRE, M.D., Professor of Orthopædic Surgery, Fractures and Dislocations, and Clinical Surgery, in Bellevue Hospital Medical College, New York. With 274 Wood Engravings, 8vo, 20s. [1876]

DISEASES OF THE RECTUM,
by THOMAS B. CURLING, F.R.S., Consulting Surgeon to the London Hospital. Fourth Edition, Revised, 8vo, 7s. 6d. [1876]

BY THE SAME AUTHOR,
DISEASES OF THE TESTIS, SPERMATIC CORD, AND SCROTUM.
Third Edition, with Engravings, 8vo, 16s. [1878]

FISTULA, HÆMORRHOIDS, PAINFUL ULCER, STRICTURE,
Prolapsus, and other Diseases of the Rectum: their Diagnosis and Treatment. By WILLIAM ALLINGHAM, F.R.C.S., Surgeon to St. Mark's Hospital for Fistula. Third Edition, with Engravings, 8vo, 10s. [1879]

HYDROCELE:
its several Varieties and their Treatment, by SAMUEL OSBORN, F.R.C.S., late Surgical Registrar to St. Thomas's Hospital. With Engravings, fcap. 8vo, 3s. [1878]

PRACTICAL LITHOTOMY AND LITHOTRITY;
or, An Inquiry into the best Modes of removing Stone from the Bladder. By Sir HENRY THOMPSON, F.R.C.S., Emeritus Professor of Surgery to University College. Second Edition, 8vo, with numerous Engravings, 10s. [1871]

BY THE SAME AUTHOR,
DISEASES OF THE URINARY ORGANS:
(Clinical Lectures). Fifth Edition, 8vo, with 2 Plates and 71 Engravings, 10s. 6d. [1879]

ALSO,
DISEASES OF THE PROSTATE:
their Pathology and Treatment. Fourth Edition, 8vo, with numerous Plates, 10s. [1873]

ALSO,
THE PREVENTIVE TREATMENT OF CALCULOUS DISEASE
and the Use of Solvent Remedies. Second Edition, fcap. 8vo, 2s. 6d. [1876]

STRICTURE OF THE URETHRA,
and other Diseases of the Urinary Organs, by REGINALD HARRISON, F.R.C.S., Surgeon to the Liverpool Royal Infirmary. With 10 plates. 8vo, 7s. 6d. [1878]

LITHOTOMY AND EXTRACTION OF STONE
from the Bladder, Urethra, and Prostate of the Male, and from the Bladder of the Female, by W. POULETT HARRIS, M.D., Surgeon-Major H.M. Bengal Medical Service. With Engravings, 8vo, 10s. 6d. [1876]

THE SURGERY OF THE RECTUM:
Lettsomian Lectures by HENRY SMITH, F.R.C.S., Professor of Surgery in King's College, Surgeon to King's College Hospital. Fourth Edition, fcap. 8vo, 5s. [1876]

DISEASES OF THE BLADDER,
Prostate Gland and Urethra, including a practical view of Urinary Diseases, Deposits and Calculi, by F. J. GANT, F.R.C.S., Senior Surgeon to the Royal Free Hospital. Fourth Edition, crown 8vo, with Engravings, 10s. 6d. [1876]

THE DIAGNOSIS OF DISEASES OF THE KIDNEYS,
with Aids thereto, by W. R. BASHAM, M.D., F.R.C.P., late Senior Physician to the Westminster Hospital. 8vo, with 10 Plates, 5s. [1872]

RENAL AND URINARY DISEASES:
Clinical Reports, by WILLIAM CARTER, M.B., M.R.C.P., Physician to the Liverpool Southern Hospital. Crown 8vo, 7s. 6d. [1878]

THE REPRODUCTIVE ORGANS
in Childhood, Youth, Adult Age, and Advanced Life (Functions and Disorders of), considered in their Physiological, Social, and Moral Relations, by WILLIAM ACTON, M.R.C.S. Sixth Edition, 8vo, 12s. [1875]

URINARY AND REPRODUCTIVE ORGANS:
their Functional Diseases, by D. CAMPBELL BLACK, M.D., L.R.C.S. Edin. Second Edition. 8vo, 10s. 6d. [1875]

LECTURES ON SYPHILIS,
and on some forms of Local Disease, affecting principally the Organs of Generation, by HENRY LEE, F.R.C.S., Surgeon to St. George's Hospital. With Engravings, 8vo, 10s. [1875]

SYPHILITIC NERVOUS AFFECTIONS:
Their Clinical Aspects, by THOMAS BUZZARD, M.D., F.R.C.P. Lond., Physician to the National Hospital for Paralysis and Epilepsy. Post 8vo, 5s. [1874]

SYPHILIS:
Harveian Lectures, by J. R. LANE, F.R.C.S., Surgeon to, and Lecturer on Surgery at, St. Mary's Hospital; Consulting Surgeon to the Lock Hospital. Fcap. 8vo, 3s. 6d. [1878]

THE MARRIAGE OF NEAR KIN,
Considered with respect to the Laws of Nations, Results of Experience, and the Teachings of Biology, by ALFRED H. HUTH. 8vo, 14s. [1875]

PATHOLOGY OF THE URINE,
including a Complete Guide to its Analysis, by J. L. W. THUDICHUM, M.D., F.R.C.P. Second Edition, rewritten and enlarged, with Engravings, 8vo, 15s. [1877]

GENITO-URINARY ORGANS, INCLUDING SYPHILIS:
A Practical Treatise on their Surgical Diseases, designed as a Manual for Students and Practitioners, by W. H. VAN BUREN, M.D., Professor of the Principles of Surgery in Bellevue Hospital Medical College, New York, and E. L. KEYES, M.D., Professor of Dermatology in Bellevue Hospital Medical College, New York. Royal 8vo, with 140 Engravings, 21s. [1874]

HISTOLOGY AND HISTO-CHEMISTRY OF MAN:
A Treatise on the Elements of Composition and Structure of the Human Body, by HEINRICH FREY, Professor of Medicine in Zurich. Translated from the Fourth German Edition by ARTHUR E. J. BARKER, Assistant-Surgeon to University College Hospital. And Revised by the Author. 8vo, with 608 Engravings, 21s. [1874]

HUMAN PHYSIOLOGY:
A Treatise designed for the Use of Students and Practitioners of Medicine, by JOHN C. DALTON, M.D., Professor of Physiology and Hygiene in the College of Physicians and Surgeons, New York. Sixth Edition, royal 8vo, with 316 Engravings, 20s. [1875]

HANDBOOK FOR THE PHYSIOLOGICAL LABORATORY,
by E. KLEIN, M.D., F.R.S., Assistant Professor in the Pathological Laboratory of the Brown Institution, London; J. BURDON-SANDERSON, M.D., F.R.S., Professor of Practical Physiology in University College, London; MICHAEL FOSTER, M.D., F.R.S., Prælector of Physiology in Trinity College, Cambridge; and T. LAUDER BRUNTON, M.D., F.R.S., Lecturer on Materia Medica at St. Bartholomew's Hospital; edited by J. BURDON-SANDERSON. 8vo, with 123 Plates, 24s. [1873]

PRACTICAL HISTOLOGY:
By WILLIAM RUTHERFORD, M.D., Professor of the Institutes of Medicine in the University of Edinburgh. Second Edition, with 63 Engravings. Crown 8vo (with additional leaves for notes), 6s. [1876]

MANUAL OF ANTHROPOMETRY:
A Guide to the Measurement of the Human Body, containing an Anthropometrical Chart and Register, a Systematic Table of Measurements, &c. By CHARLES ROBERTS, F.R.C.S., late Assistant Surgeon to the Victoria Hospital for Children. With numerous Illustrations and Tables. 8vo, 6s. 6d. [1878]

PRINCIPLES OF HUMAN PHYSIOLOGY,
by W. B. CARPENTER, C.B., M.D., F.R.S. Eighth Edition by HENRY POWER, M.B., F.R.C.S., Examiner in Natural Science, University of Oxford, and in Natural Science and Medicine, University of Cambridge. 8vo, with 3 Steel Plates and 371 Engravings, 31s. 6d. [1876]

STUDENTS' GUIDE TO HUMAN OSTEOLOGY,
By WILLIAM WARWICK WAGSTAFFE, F.R.C.S., Assistant-Surgeon and Lecturer on Anatomy, St. Thomas's Hospital. With 23 Plates and 66 Engravings. Fcap. 8vo, 10s. 6d. [1875]

LANDMARKS, MEDICAL AND SURGICAL,
By LUTHER HOLDEN, F.R.C.S., Member of the Court of Examiners of the Royal College of Surgeons. Second Edition, 8vo, 3s. 6d. [1877]

BY THE SAME AUTHOR.

HUMAN OSTEOLOGY:
Comprising a Description of the Bones, with Delineations of the Attachments of the Muscles, the General and Microscopical Structure of Bone, and its Development. Fifth Edition, with 61 Lithographic Plates and 89 Engravings. 8vo, 16s. [1878]

PATHOLOGICAL ANATOMY:
Lectures by SAMUEL WILKS, M.D., F.R.S., Physician to, and Lecturer on Medicine at, Guy's Hospital; and WALTER MOXON, M.D., F.R.C.P., Physician to, and Lecturer on Materia Medica at, Guy's Hospital. Second Edition, 8vo, with Plates, 18s. [1875]

PATHOLOGICAL ANATOMY·
A Manual by C. HANDFIELD JONES, M.B., F.R.S., Physician to St. Mary's Hospital, and EDWARD H. SIEVEKING, M.D., F.R.C.P., Physician to St. Mary's Hospital. Edited by J. F. PAYNE, M.D., F.R.C.P., Assistant Physician and Lecturer on General Pathology at St. Thomas's Hospital. Second Edition, crown 8vo, with 195 Engravings, 16s. [1875]

POST-MORTEM EXAMINATIONS:
a Description and Explanation of the Method of Performing them, with especial Reference to Medico-Legal Practice. By Professor RUDOLPH VIRCHOW, of Berlin. Fcap 8vo, 2s. 6d. [1876]

STUDENT'S GUIDE TO SURGICAL ANATOMY:
a Text-book for the Pass Examination, by E. BELLAMY, F.R.C.S., Surgeon and Lecturer on Anatomy at Charing Cross Hospital. Fcap 8vo, with 50 Engravings, 6s. 6d. [1873]

ANATOMY OF THE JOINTS OF MAN,
by HENRY MORRIS, F.R.C.S., Surgeon to, and Lecturer on Anatomy and Demonstrator of Operative Surgery at, the Middlesex Hospital. With 44 Lithographic Plates (several being coloured) and 13 Wood Engravings. 8vo, 16s. [1879]

MEDICAL ANATOMY,
by FRANCIS SIBSON, M.D., F.R.C.P., F.R.S. Imp. folio, with 21 coloured Plates, cloth, 42s., half-morocco, 50s. [1869]

PRACTICAL ANATOMY:
a Manual of Dissections by CHRISTOPHER HEATH, F.R.C.S., Surgeon to University College Hospital, and Holme Professor of Surgery in University College. Fourth Edition, crown 8vo, with 16 Coloured Plates and 264 Engravings, 14s. [1877]

AN ATLAS OF HUMAN ANATOMY:
illustrating most of the ordinary Dissections, and many not usually practised by the Student. To be completed in 12 or 13 Bi-monthly Parts, each containing 4 Coloured Plates, with Explanatory Text. By RICKMAN J. GODLEE, M.S., F.R.C.S., Assistant Surgeon to University College Hospital, and Senior Demonstrator of Anatomy in University College. Parts I to VII. Imp. 4to, 7s. 6d. each Part. [1877-9]

THE ANATOMIST'S VADE-MECUM:
a System of Human Anatomy by ERASMUS WILSON, F.R.C.S., F.R.S. Ninth Edition, by G. BUCHANAN, M.A., M.D., Professor of Clinical Surgery in the University of Glasgow, and HENRY E. CLARK, F.F.P.S., Lecturer on Anatomy at the Glasgow Royal Infirmary School of Medicine. Crown 8vo, with 371 Engravings, 14s. [1873]

ATLAS OF TOPOGRAPHICAL ANATOMY,
after Plane Sections of Frozen Bodies. By WILHELM BRAUNE, Professor of Anatomy in the University of Leipzig. Translated by EDWARD BELLAMY, F.R.C.S., Surgeon to, and Lecturer on Anatomy, &c., at, Charing Cross Hospital. With 34 Photo-lithographic Plates and 46 Woodcuts. Large Imp. 8vo, 40s. [1877]

THE ANATOMICAL REMEMBRANCER;
or, Complete Pocket Anatomist. Eighth Edition, 32mo, 3s. 6d. [1876]

THE STUDENT'S GUIDE TO THE PRACTICE OF MEDICINE,
by MATTHEW CHARTERIS, M.D., Professor of Medicine in Anderson's College, and Lecturer on Clinical Medicine in the Royal Infirmary, Glasgow. Second Edition, with Engravings on Copper and Wood, fcap. 8vo, 6s. 6d. [1878]

THE MICROSCOPE IN MEDICINE,
by LIONEL S. BEALE, M.B., F.R.S., Physician to King's College Hospital. Fourth Edition, with 86 Plates, 8vo, 21s. [1877]

HOOPER'S PHYSICIAN'S VADE-MECUM;
or, Manual of the Principles and Practice of Physic, Ninth Edition by W. A. GUY, M.B., F.R.S., and JOHN HARLEY, M.D., F.R.C.P. Fcap 8vo, with Engravings, 12s. 6d. [1874]

A NEW SYSTEM OF MEDICINE;
entitled Recognisant Medicine, or the State of the Sick, by BHOLANOTH BOSE, M.D., Indian Medical Service. 8vo, 10s. 6d. [1877]

BY THE SAME AUTHOR.

PRINCIPLES OF RATIONAL THERAPEUTICS.
Commenced as an Inquiry into the Relative Value of Quinine and Arsenic in Ague. 8vo, 4s. [1877]

THE STUDENT'S GUIDE TO MEDICAL DIAGNOSIS,
by SAMUEL FENWICK, M.D., F.R.C.P., Physician to the London Hospital. Fourth Edition, fcap. 8vo, with 106 Engravings, 6s. 6d. [1876]

A MANUAL OF MEDICAL DIAGNOSIS,
by A. W. BARCLAY, M.D., F.R.C.P., Physician to, and Lecturer on Medicine at, St. George's Hospital. Third Edition, fcap 8vo, 10s. 6d. [1876]

CLINICAL MEDICINE:
Lectures and Essays by BALTHAZAR FOSTER, M.D., F.R.C.P. Lond., Professor of Medicine in Queen's College, Birmingham. 8vo, 10s. 6d. [1874]

CLINICAL STUDIES:
Illustrated by Cases observed in Hospital and Private Practice, by Sir J. ROSE CORMACK, M.D., F.R.S.E., Physician to the Hertford British Hospital of Paris. 2 vols., post 8vo, 20s. [1876]

CLINICAL REMINISCENCES:
By PEYTON BLAKISTON, M.D., F.R.S. Post 8vo, 3s. 6d. [1878]

ROYLE'S MANUAL OF MATERIA MEDICA AND THERAPEUTICS.
Sixth Edition by JOHN HARLEY, M.D., F.R.C.P., Physician to, and Joint Lecturer on Clinical Medicine at, St. Thomas's Hospital. Crown 8vo, with 139 Engravings, 15s. [1876]

PRACTICAL THERAPEUTICS:
A Manual by E. J. WARING, M.D., F.R.C.P. Lond. Third Edition, fcap 8vo, 12s. 6d. [1871]

THE ELEMENTS OF THERAPEUTICS.
A Clinical Guide to the Action of Drugs, by C. BINZ, M.D., Professor of Pharmacology in the University of Bonn. Translated and Edited with Additions, in Conformity with the British and American Pharmacopœias, by EDWARD I. SPARKS, F.R.C.P., M.A., M.B. Oxon., formerly Radcliffe Travelling Fellow. Crown 8vo, 8s. 6d. [1877]

THE STUDENT'S GUIDE TO MATERIA MEDICA,
by JOHN C. THOROWGOOD, M.D., F.R.C.P. Lond., Physician to the City of London Hospital for Diseases of the Chest. Fcap 8vo, with Engravings, 6s. 6d. [1874]

THE NATIONAL DISPENSATORY
containing the Natural History, Chemistry, Pharmacy, Actions and Uses of Medicines, including those recognised in the Pharmacopœias of the United States and Great Britain, by ALFRED STILLÉ, M.D., LL.D., and JOHN M. MAISCH, Ph.D., with 201 Engravings, 1628 pp., 8vo., 34s. [1879]

DENTAL MATERIA MEDICA AND THERAPEUTICS,
Elements of, by JAMES STOCKEN, L.D.S.R.C.S., Lecturer on Dental Materia Medica and Therapeutics to the National Dental Hospital. Second Edition, Fcap 8vo, 6s. 6d. [1878]

THE DISEASES OF CHILDREN:
A Practical Manual, with a Formulary, by EDWARD ELLIS, M.D., late Senior Physician to the Victoria Hospital for Children. Third Edition, crown 8vo, 7s. 6d. [1876]

THE WASTING DISEASES OF CHILDREN,
by EUSTACE SMITH, M.D., F.R.C.P. Lond., Physician to the King of the Belgians, Physician to the East London Hospital for Children. Third Edition, post 8vo, 8s. 6d. [1876]

BY THE SAME AUTHOR,
CLINICAL STUDIES OF DISEASE IN CHILDREN.
Post 8vo, 7s. 6d. [1876]

INFANT FEEDING AND ITS INFLUENCE ON LIFE;
or, the Causes and Prevention of Infant Mortality, by CHARLES H. F. ROUTH, M.D., Senior Physician to the Samaritan Hospital for Women and Children. Third Edition, fcap 8vo, 7s. 6d. [1876]

COMPENDIUM OF CHILDREN'S DISEASES:
A Handbook for Practitioners and Students, by JOHANN STEINER, M.D., Professor in the University of Prague. Translated from the Second German Edition by LAWSON TAIT, F.R.C.S., Surgeon to the Birmingham Hospital for Women. 8vo, 12s. 6d. [1874]

THE DISEASES OF CHILDREN:
Essays by WILLIAM HENRY DAY, M.D., Physician to the Samaritan Hospital for Diseases of Women and Children. Second Edition, fcap 8vo.
[In the Press.]

PUERPERAL DISEASES:
Clinical Lectures by FORDYCE BARKER, M.D., Obstetric Physician to Bellevue Hospital, New York. 8vo, 15s. [1874]

THE STUDENT'S GUIDE TO THE PRACTICE OF MIDWIFERY, by D. LLOYD ROBERTS, M.D., F.R.C.P., Physician to St. Mary's Hospital, Manchester. Second Edition, fcap. 8vo, with 96 Engravings, 7s.
[1879]

OBSTETRIC MEDICINE AND SURGERY,
Their Principles and Practice, by F. H. RAMSBOTHAM, M.D., F.R.C.P. Fifth Edition, 8vo, with 120 Plates, 22s. [1867]

OBSTETRIC SURGERY:
A Complete Handbook, giving Short Rules of Practice in every Emergency, from the Simplest to the most Formidable Operations connected with the Science of Obstetricy, by CHARLES CLAY, Ext.L.R.C.P. Lond., L.R.C.S.E., late Senior Surgeon and Lecturer on Midwifery, St. Mary's Hospital, Manchester. Fcap 8vo, with 91 Engravings, 6s. 6d.
[1874]

SCHROEDER'S MANUAL OF MIDWIFERY,
including the Pathology of Pregnancy and the Puerperal State. Translated by CHARLES H. CARTER, B.A., M.D. 8vo, with Engravings, 12s. 6d. [1873]

OBSTETRIC OPERATIONS,
  including the Treatment of Hæmorrhage, and forming a Guide to the Management of Difficult Labour; Lectures by ROBERT BARNES, M.D., F.R.C.P., Obstetric Physician to St. George's Hospital. Third Edition, 8vo, with 124 Engravings, 18s. [1876]

BY THE SAME AUTHOR,
MEDICAL AND SURGICAL DISEASES OF WOMEN:
  a Clinical History. Second Edition, 8vo, with 181 Engravings, 28s. [1878]

LECTURES ON THE DISEASES OF WOMEN,
  by CHARLES WEST, M.D., F.R.C.P. Fourth Edition, Revised and in part Re-written by the Author, with numerous Additions by J. MATTHEWS DUNCAN, M.D., Obstetric Physician to St. Bartholomew's Hospital. 8vo, 16s. [1879]

THE PRINCIPLES AND PRACTICE OF GYNÆCOLOGY,
  by THOMAS ADDIS EMMET, M.D., Surgeon to the Woman's Hospital of the State of New York. With 130 Engravings, royal 8vo, 24s. [1879]

THE STUDENT'S GUIDE TO THE DISEASES OF WOMEN,
  by ALFRED L. GALABIN, M.D., F.R.C.P., Assistant Obstetric Physician to Guy's Hospital. With 63 Engravings, fcap. 8vo, 7s. 6d. [1879]

OBSTETRIC APHORISMS:
  for the Use of Students commencing Midwifery Practice, by J. G. SWAYNE, M.D., Consulting Physician-Accoucheur to the Bristol General Hospital. Sixth Edition, fcap. 8vo, with Engravings, 3s. 6d. [1876]

A HANDBOOK OF UTERINE THERAPEUTICS,
  and of Diseases of Women, by E. J. TILT, M.D., M.R.C.P. Fourth Edition, post 8vo, 10s. [1878]

BY THE SAME AUTHOR,
THE CHANGE OF LIFE
  in Health and Disease: a Practical Treatise on the Nervous and other Affections incidental to Women at the Decline of Life. Third Edition, 8vo, 10s. 6d. [1870]

DISEASES OF THE OVARIES:
  their Diagnosis and Treatment, by T. SPENCER WELLS, F.R.C.S., Surgeon to the Queen's Household and to the Samaritan Hospital. 8vo, with about 150 Engravings, 21s. [1872]

PRACTICAL GYNÆCOLOGY:
  A Handbook of the Diseases of Women, by HEYWOOD SMITH, M.D. Oxon., Physician to the Hospital for Women and to the British Lying-in Hospital. With Engravings, crown 8vo, 5s. 6d. [1877]

RUPTURE OF THE FEMALE PERINEUM,
  Its treatment, immediate and remote, by GEORGE G. BANTOCK, M.D., Surgeon (for In-patients) to the Samaritan Free Hospital for Women and Children. With 2 plates, 8vo, 3s. 6d. [1878

PAPERS ON THE FEMALE PERINEUM, &c.,
by JAMES MATTHEWS DUNCAN, M.D., Obstetric Physician to St. Bartholomew's Hospital. 8vo, 6s. [1878]

INFLUENCE OF POSTURE ON WOMEN
In Gynecic and Obstetric Practice, by J. H. AVELING, M.D., Physician to the Chelsea Hospital for Women, Vice-President of the Obstetrical Society of London. 8vo, 6s. [1878]

A MANUAL FOR HOSPITAL NURSES
and others engaged in Attending on the Sick by EDWARD J. DOMVILLE, L.R.C.P., M.R.C.S., Surgeon to the Exeter Lying-in Charity. Third Edition, crown 8vo, 2s. 6d. [1878]

THE NURSE'S COMPANION:
A Manual of General and Monthly Nursing, by CHARLES J. CULLINGWORTH, Surgeon to St. Mary's Hospital, Manchester. Fcap. 8vo, 2s. 6d. [1876]

LECTURES ON NURSING,
by WILLIAM ROBERT SMITH, M.B., Honorary Medical Officer, Hospital for Sick Children, Sheffield. Second Edition, with 26 Engravings. Post 8vo, 6s. [1878]

HANDBOOK FOR NURSES FOR THE SICK,
by ZEPHERINA P. VEITCH. Second Edition, crown 8vo, 3s. 6d. [1876]

A COMPENDIUM OF DOMESTIC MEDICINE
and Companion to the Medicine Chest; intended as a Source of Easy Reference for Clergymen, and for Families residing at a Distance from Professional Assistance, by JOHN SAVORY, M.S.A. Ninth Edition, 12mo, 5s. [1878]

HOSPITAL MORTALITY
being a Statistical Investigation of the Returns of the Hospitals of Great Britain and Ireland for fifteen years, by LAWSON TAIT, F.R.C.S., F.S.S. 8vo, 8s. 6d. [1877]

THE COTTAGE HOSPITAL:
Its Origin, Progress, Management, and Work, by HENRY C. BURDETT, the Seaman's Hospital, Greenwich. With Engravings, crown 8vo, 7s. 6d. [1877]

WINTER COUGH:
(Catarrh, Bronchitis, Emphysema, Asthma), Lectures by HORACE DOBELL, M.D., Consulting Physician to the Royal Hospital for Diseases of the Chest. Third Edition, with Coloured Plates, 8vo, 10s. 6d. [1875]

BY THE SAME AUTHOR,
LOSS OF WEIGHT, BLOOD-SPITTING, AND LUNG DISEASE.
With Chromo-lithograph, 8vo, 10s. 6d. [1878]

INJURIES AND DISEASES OF THE LYMPHATIC SYSTEM,
by S. MESSENGER BRADLEY, F.R.C.S., Lecturer on Practical Surgery in Owen's College, Manchester. 8vo., 5s. [1879]

CONSUMPTION:
Its Nature, Symptoms, Causes, Prevention, Curability, and Treatment. By PETER GOWAN, M.D., B. Sc., late Physician and Surgeon in Ordinary to the King of Siam. Crown 8vo. 5s. [1878]

NOTES ON ASTHMA;
its Forms and Treatment, by JOHN C. THOROWGOOD, M.D. Lond., F.R.C.P., Physician to the Hospital for Diseases of the Chest, Victoria Park. Third Edition, crown 8vo, 4s. 6d. [1878]

ASTHMA
Its Pathology and Treatment, by J. B. BERKART, M.D., Assistant Physician to the City of London Hospital for Diseases of the Chest. 8vo, 7s. 6d. [1878]

PROGNOSIS IN CASES OF VALVULAR DISEASE OF THE
Heart, by THOMAS B. PEACOCK, M.D., F.R.C.P., Honorary Consulting Physician to St. Thomas's Hospital. 8vo, 3s. 6d. [1877]

DISEASES OF THE HEART:
Their Pathology, Diagnosis, Prognosis, and Treatment (a Manual), by ROBERT H. SEMPLE, M.D., F.R.C.P., Physician to the Hospital for Diseases of the Throat. 8vo, 8s. 6d. [1875]

CHRONIC DISEASE OF THE HEART:
Its Bearings upon Pregnancy, Parturition and Childbed. By ANGUS MACDONALD, M.D., F.R.S.E., Physician to, and Clinical Lecturer on the Diseases of Women at, the Edinburgh Royal Infirmary. With Engravings, 8vo, 8s. 6d. [1875]

PHTHISIS:
In a series of Clinical Studies, by AUSTIN FLINT, M.D., Professor of the Principles and Practice of Medicine and of Clinical Medicine in the Bellevue Hospital Medical College. 8vo, 16s. [1875]

BY THE SAME AUTHOR,

A MANUAL OF PERCUSSION AND AUSCULTATION,
of the Physical Diagnosis of Diseases of the Lungs and Heart, and of Thoracic Aneurism. Post 8vo, 6s. 6d. [1876]

DIPHTHERIA:
its Nature and Treatment, Varieties, and Local Expressions, by MORELL MACKENZIE, M.D., Physician to the Hospital for Diseases of the Throat. Crown 8vo, 5s. [1878]

DISEASES OF THE HEART AND AORTA,
By THOMAS HAYDEN, F.K.Q.C.P. Irel., Physician to the Mater Misericordiæ Hospital, Dublin. With 80 Engravings. 8vo, 25s. [1875]

DISEASES OF THE HEART
and of the Lungs in Connexion therewith—Notes and Observations by THOMAS SHAPTER, M.D., F.R.C.P. Lond., Senior Physician to the Devon and Exeter Hospital. 8vo, 7s. 6d. [1874]

DISEASES OF THE HEART AND AORTA:
Clinical Lectures by GEORGE W. BALFOUR, M.D., F.R.C.P., Physician to, and Lecturer on Clinical Medicine in, the Royal Infirmary, Edinburgh. 8vo, with Engravings, 12s. 6d. [1876]

PHYSICAL DIAGNOSIS OF DISEASES OF THE HEART.
Lectures by ARTHUR E. SANSOM, M.D., F.R.C.P., Assistant Physician to the London Hospital. Second Edition, with Engravings, fcap. 8vo, 4s. 6d. [1876]

TRACHEOTOMY,
especially in Relation to Diseases of the Larynx and Trachea, by PUGIN THORNTON, M.R.C.S., late Surgeon to the Hospital for Diseases of the Throat. With Photographic Plates and Woodcuts, 8vo, 5s. 6d. [1876]

SORE THROAT:
Its Nature, Varieties, and Treatment, including the Connexion between Affections of the Throat and other Diseases. By PROSSER JAMES, M.D., Lecturer on Materia Medica and Therapeutics at the London Hospital, Physician to the Hospital for Diseases of the Throat. Third Edition, with Coloured Plates, 5s. 6d. [1878]

LECTURES ON SYPHILIS OF THE LARYNX
(Lesions of the Secondary and Intermediate Stages), by W. MACNEILL WHISTLER, M.D., Physician to the Hospital for Diseases of the Throat and Chest. Post 8vo, 4s. [1879]

WINTER AND SPRING
on the Shores of the Mediterranean. By HENRY BENNET, M.D. Fifth Edition, post 8vo, with numerous Plates, Maps, and Engravings, 12s. 6d. [1874]

BY THE SAME AUTHOR,
TREATMENT OF PULMONARY CONSUMPTION
by Hygiene, Climate, and Medicine. Third Edition, 8vo, 7s. 6d. [1878]

PRINCIPAL HEALTH RESORTS
of Europe and Africa, and their Use in the Treatment of Chronic Diseases. A Handbook by THOMAS MORE MADDEN, M.D., M.R.I.A., Vice-President of the Dublin Obstetrical Society. 8vo, 10s. [1876]

THE BATH THERMAL WATERS:
Historical, Social, and Medical, by JOHN KENT SPENDER, M.D., Surgeon to the Mineral Water Hospital, Bath. With an Appendix on the Climate of Bath by the Rev. L. BLOMEFIELD, M.A., F.L.S., F.G.S. 8vo, 7s. 6d. [1877]

THE BATH WATERS:
Their Uses and Effects in the Cure and Relief of various Chronic Diseases. By JAMES TUNSTALL, M.D. Fifth Edition, revised, and in part re-written, by RICHARD CARTER, M.D., Surgeon to the Bath Mineral Hospital. Post 8vo, 2s. 6d. [1879]

ENDEMIC DISEASES OF TROPICAL CLIMATES,
with their Treatment, by JOHN SULLIVAN, M.D., M.R.C.P. Post 8vo, 6s. [1877]

DISEASES OF TROPICAL CLIMATES
and their Treatment: with Hints for the Preservation of Health in the Tropics, by JAMES A. HORTON, M.D., Surgeon-Major, Army Medical Department. Second Edition, post 8vo, 12s. 6d. [1879]

HEALTH IN INDIA FOR BRITISH WOMEN
and on the Prevention of Disease in Tropical Climates by EDWARD J. TILT, M.D. Fourth Edition, crown 8vo, 5s. [1875]

BAZAAR MEDICINES OF INDIA
and Common Medical Plants: Remarks on their Uses, with Full Index of Diseases, indicating their Treatment by these and other Agents procurable throughout India, &c., by EDWARD J. WARING, M.D., F.R.C.P. Third Edition. Fcap 8vo, 5s. [1875]

SOME AFFECTIONS OF THE LIVER
and Intestinal Canal; with Remarks on Ague and its Sequelæ, Scurvy, Purpura, &c., by STEPHEN H. WARD, M.D. Lond., F.R.C.P., Physician to the Seamen's Hospital, Greenwich. 8vo, 7s. [1872]

DISEASES OF THE STOMACH.
The Varieties of Dyspepsia, their Diagnosis and Treatment. By S. O. HABERSHON, M.D., F.R.C.P., Senior Physician to Guy's Hospital. Third Edition, crown 8vo, 5s. [1879]

BY THE SAME AUTHOR,

PATHOLOGY OF THE PNEUMOGASTRIC NERVE,
being the Lumleian Lectures for 1876. Post 8vo, 3s. 6d. [1877]

ALSO,

DISEASES OF THE ABDOMEN,
comprising those of the Stomach and other parts of the Alimentary Canal, Œsophagus, Cæcum, Intestines, and Peritoneum. Third Edition, with 5 Plates, 8vo, 21s. [1878]

LECTURES ON DISEASES OF THE NERVOUS SYSTEM,
by SAMUEL WILKS, M.D., F.R.S., Physician to, and Lecturer on Medicine at, Guy's Hospital. 8vo, 15s. [1878]

NERVOUS DISEASES:
their Description and Treatment, by ALLEN McLANE HAMILTON, M.D., Physician at the Epileptic and Paralytic Hospital, Blackwell's Island, New York City. Roy. 8vo, with 53 Illustrations, 14s. [1878]

NUTRITION IN HEALTH AND DISEASE:
A Contribution to Hygiene and to Clinical Medicine. By HENRY BENNET, M.D. Third (Library) Edition. 8vo, 7s. Cheap Edition, Fcap. 8vo, 2s. 6d. [1877]

HEADACHES:
their Causes, Nature, and Treatment. By WILLIAM H. DAY, M.D., Physician to the Samaritan Free Hospital for Women and Children. Second Edition, crown 8vo, with Engravings. 6s. 6d. [1878]

PUBLISHED BY J. AND A. CHURCHILL

FOOD AND DIETETICS,
Physiologically and Therapeutically Considered. By FREDERICK W. PAVY, M.D., F.R.S., Physician to Guy's Hospital. Second Edition, 8vo, 15s. [1875]

BY THE SAME AUTHOR.

CERTAIN POINTS CONNECTED WITH DIABETES
(Croonian Lectures). 8vo, 4s. 6d. [1878]

IMPERFECT DIGESTION:
its Causes and Treatment by ARTHUR LEARED, M.D., F.R.C.P., Senior Physician to the Great Northern Hospital. Sixth Edition, fcap 8vo, 4s. 6d. [1875]

MEGRIM, SICK-HEADACHE,
and some Allied Disorders: a Contribution to the Pathology of Nerve-Storms, by EDWARD LIVEING, M.D. Cantab., F.R.C.P., Hon. Fellow of King's College, London. 8vo, with Coloured Plate, 15s. [1873]

THE SYMPATHETIC SYSTEM OF NERVES:
their Physiology and Pathology, by A. EULENBURG, Professor of Medicine, University of Greifswald, and Dr. P. GUTTMANN, Privat Docent in Medicine, University of Berlin. Translated by A. NAPIER, M.D., F.F.P.S 8vo, 5s. [1879]

RHEUMATIC GOUT,
or Chronic Rheumatic Arthritis of all the Joints; a Treatise by ROBERT ADAMS, M.D., M.R.I.A., late Surgeon to H.M. the Queen in Ireland, and Regius Professor of Surgery in the University of Dublin. Second Edition, 8vo, with Atlas of Plates, 21s. [1872]

GOUT, RHEUMATISM,
and the Allied Affections; with a chapter on Longevity and the Causes Antagonistic to it, by PETER HOOD, M.D. Second Edition, crown 8vo, 10s. 6d. [1879]

RHEUMATISM.
Notes by JULIUS POLLOCK, M.D., F.R.C.P., Senior Physician to, and Lecturer on Medicine at, Charing Cross Hospital. Second Edition, with Engravings, fcap. 8vo, 3s. 6d. [1879]

CERTAIN FORMS OF CANCER,
with a New and successful Mode of Treating it, to which is prefixed a Practical and Systematic Description of all the varieties of this Disease, by ALEX. MARSDEN, M.D., F.R.C.S.E., Consulting Surgeon to the Royal Free Hospital, and Senior Surgeon to the Cancer Hospital. Second Edition, with Coloured Plates, 8vo, 8s. 6d. [1873]

ATLAS OF SKIN DISEASES:
a series of Illustrations, with Descriptive Text and Notes upon Treatment. By TILBURY FOX, M.D., F.R.C.P., Physician to the Department for Skin Diseases in University College Hospital. With 72 Coloured Plates, royal 4to, half morocco, £6 6s. [1877]

LECTURES ON DERMATOLOGY;
delivered at the Royal College of Surgeons, by ERASMUS WILSON, F.R.C.S., F.R.S., 1870, 6s.; 1871-3, 10s. 6d., 1874-5, 10s. 6d.; 1876-8, 10s. 6d.

ECZEMA:
by McCALL ANDERSON, M.D., Professor of Clinical Medicine in the University of Glasgow. Third Edition, 8vo, with Engravings, 7s. 6d. [1874]

PSORIASIS OR LEPRA,
by GEORGE GASKOIN, M.R.C.S., Surgeon to the British Hospital for Diseases of the Skin. 8vo, 5s. [1875]

CERTAIN ENDEMIC SKIN AND OTHER DISEASES
of India and Hot Climates generally, by TILBURY FOX, M.D., F.R.C.P., and T. FARQUHAR, M.D. (Published under the sanction of the Secretary of State for India in Council). 8vo, 10s. 6d.

ON CERTAIN RARE DISEASES OF THE SKIN
Being vol. 1 of Lectures on Clinical Surgery. By JONATHAN HUTCHINSON, F.R.C.S., Senior Surgeon to the London Hospital, and to the Hospital for Diseases of the Skin. 8vo, 10s. 6d. [1879]

PARASITES:
a Treatise on the Entozoa of Man and Animals, including some account of the Ectozoa. By T. SPENCER COBBOLD, M.D., F.R.S., Professor of Botany and Helminthology, Royal Veterinary College. With 85 Engravings. 8vo, 15s. [1879]

MEDICAL JURISPRUDENCE,
Its Principles and Practice, by ALFRED S. TAYLOR, M.D., F.R.C.P., F.R.S. Second Edition, 2 vols., 8vo, with 189 Engravings, £1 11s. 6d. [1873]

BY THE SAME AUTHOR,

A MANUAL OF MEDICAL JURISPRUDENCE.
Tenth Edition. Crown 8vo, with 55 Engravings, 14s. [1879]

ALSO,

POISONS,
in Relation to Medical Jurisprudence and Medicine. Third Edition, crown 8vo, with 104 Engravings, 16s. [1875]

MEDICAL JURISPRUDENCE:
Lectures by FRANCIS OGSTON, M.D., Professor of Medical Jurisprudence and Medical Logic in the University of Aberdeen. Edited by FRANCIS OGSTON, Jun., M.D., Assistant to the Professor of Medical Jurisprudence and Lecturer on Practical Toxicology in the University of Aberdeen. 8vo, with 12 Copper Plates, 18s. [1878]

IDIOCY AND IMBECILITY,
by WILLIAM W. IRELAND, M.D., Medical Superintendent of the Scottish National Institution for the Education of Imbecile Children at Larbert, Stirlingshire. With Engravings, 8vo, 14s. [1877]

A MANUAL OF PSYCHOLOGICAL MEDICINE:
containing the Lunacy Laws, Nosology, Ætiology, Statistics, Description, Diagnosis, Pathology, and Treatment of Insanity, with an Appendix of Cases. By JOHN C. BUCKNILL, M.D., F.R.S., and D. HACK TUKE, M.D., F.R.C.P. Fourth Edition, with 12 Plates (30 Figures) and Engravings. 8vo, 25s. [1879]

A HANDY-BOOK OF FORENSIC MEDICINE AND TOXICOLOGY,
by W. BATHURST WOODMAN, M.D., F.R.C.P., Assistant Physician and Co-Lecturer on Physiology and Histology at the London Hospital; and C. MEYMOTT TIDY, M.D., F.C.S., Professor of Chemistry and of Medical Jurisprudence and Public Health at the London Hospital. With 8 Lithographic Plates and 116 Engravings, 8vo, 31s. 6d. [1877]

MEDICAL OPHTHALMOSCOPY:
A Manual and Atlas, by WILLIAM R. GOWERS, M.D., F.R.C.P., Assistant Professor of Medicine in University College, and Assistant Physician to the Hospital. With 16 Coloured Autotype and Lithographic Plates, and Woodcuts, comprising 112 Original Illustrations of the Changes in the Eye in Diseases of the Brain, Kidneys, &c. 8vo, 18s. [1879]

THE MEDICAL ADVISER IN LIFE ASSURANCE,
by EDWARD HENRY SIEVEKING, M.D., F.R.C.P., Physician to St. Mary's and the Lock Hospitals; Physician-Extraordinary to the Queen; Physician-in-Ordinary to the Prince of Wales, &c. Crown 8vo, 6s. [1874]

MADNESS:
in its Medical, Legal, and Social Aspects, Lectures by EDGAR SHEPPARD, M.D., M.R.C.P., Professor of Psychological Medicine in King's College; one of the Medical Superintendents of the Colney Hatch Lunatic Asylum. 8vo, 6s. 6d. [1873]

A MANUAL OF PRACTICAL HYGIENE,
by E. A. PARKES, M.D., F.R.S. Fifth Edition, by F. DE CHAUMONT, M.D., F.R.S., Professor of Military Hygiene in the Army Medical School. 8vo, with 9 Plates and 112 Engravings, 18s. [1878]

SANITARY EXAMINATIONS
of Water, Air, and Food. A Vade Mecum for the Medical Officer of Health, by CORNELIUS B. FOX, M.D. With 94 Engravings, crown 8vo, 12s. 6d. [1878]

DANGERS TO HEALTH:
A Pictorial Guide to Domestic Sanitary Defects, by T. PRIDGIN TEALE, M.A., Surgeon to the Leeds General Infirmary. With 55 Lithographs, 8vo, 10s. [1878]

MICROSCOPICAL EXAMINATION OF DRINKING WATER:
A Guide, by JOHN D. MACDONALD, M.D., F.R.S., Assistant Professor of Naval Hygiene, Army Medical School. 8vo, with 24 Plates, 7s. 6d. [1875]

A HANDBOOK OF HYGIENE AND SANITARY SCIENCE,
 by GEORGE WILSON, M.A., M.D., Medical Officer of Health for Mid-Warwickshire. Third Edition, post 8vo, with Engravings, 10s. 6d.
 [1677]
HANDBOOK OF MEDICAL AND SURGICAL ELECTRICITY,
 by HERBERT TIBBITS, M.D., F.R.C.P.E., Senior Physician to the West London Hospital for Paralysis and Epilepsy. Second Edition, 8vo, with 95 Engravings, 9s. [1877]
BY THE SAME AUTHOR.
A MAP OF ZIEMSSEN'S MOTOR POINTS OF THE HUMAN BODY·
 a Guide to Localised Electrisation. Mounted on Rollers, 35 × 21. With 20 Illustrations, 5s. [1877]
CLINICAL USES OF ELECTRICITY;
 Lectures delivered at University College Hospital by J. RUSSELL REYNOLDS, M.D. Lond., F.R.C.P., F.R.S., Professor of Medicine in University College. Second Edition, post 8vo, 3s. 6d. [1873]
MEDICO-ELECTRIC APPARATUS:
 A Practical Description of every Form in Modern Use, with Plain Directions for Mounting, Charging, and Working, by SALT & SON, Birmingham. Second Edition, revised and enlarged, with 33 Engravings, 8vo, 2s. 6d. [1877]
A DICTIONARY OF MEDICAL SCIENCE;
 containing a concise explanation of the various subjects and terms of Medicine, &c.; Notices of Climate and Mineral Waters; Formulæ for Officinal, Empirical, and Dietetic Preparations; with the Accentuation and Etymology of the terms and the French and other Synonyms, by ROBLEY DUNGLISON, M.D., LL.D. New Edition, royal 8vo, 28s. [1874]
A MEDICAL VOCABULARY;
 being an Explanation of all Terms and Phrases used in the various Departments of Medical Science and Practice, giving their derivation, meaning, application, and pronunciation, by ROBERT G. MAYNE, M.D., LL.D. Fourth Edition, fcap 8vo, 10s. [1875]
DISEASES OF THE EYE:
 a Manual by C. MACNAMARA, F.R.C.S., Surgeon to Westminster Hospital. Third Edition, fcap. 8vo, with Coloured Plates and Engravings, 12s. 6d. [1876]
DISEASES OF THE EYE:
 A Practical Treatise by HAYNES WALTON, F.R.C.S., Surgeon to St. Mary's Hospital and in charge of its Ophthalmological Department. Third Edition, 8vo, with 3 Plates and nearly 300 Engravings, 25s.
 [1875]
HINTS ON OPHTHALMIC OUT-PATIENT PRACTICE,
 by CHARLES HIGGENS, F.R.C.S., Ophthalmic Assistant Surgeon to, and Lecturer on Ophthalmology at, Guy's Hospital. Second Edition, fcap. 8vo, 3s. [1879]

DISEASES OF THE EYE:
A Treatise by J. SOELBERG WELLS, F.R.C.S., Ophthalmic Surgeon to King's College Hospital and Surgeon to the Royal London Ophthalmic Hospital. Third Edition, 8vo, with Coloured Plates and Engravings, 25s. [1873]

BY THE SAME AUTHOR,
LONG, SHORT, AND WEAK SIGHT,
and their Treatment by the Scientific use of Spectacles. Fourth Edition, 8vo, 6s. [1873]

ESSAYS IN OPHTHALMOLOGY,
by GEORGE E. WALKER, F.R.C.S., Surgeon to St. Paul's Eye and Ear Hospital, &c., Liverpool. Post 8vo, 6s. [1879]

A SYSTEM OF DENTAL SURGERY,
by JOHN TOMES, F.R.S., and CHARLES S. TOMES, M.A., F.R.S., Lecturer on Dental Anatomy and Physiology at the Dental Hospital of London. Second Edition, fcap 8vo, with 268 Engravings, 14s. [1873]

DENTAL ANATOMY, HUMAN AND COMPARATIVE:
A Manual, by CHARLES S. TOMES, M.A., F.R.S., Lecturer on Dental Anatomy and Physiology at the Dental Hospital of London. With 179 Engravings, crown 8vo, 10s. 6d. [1876]

A MANUAL OF DENTAL MECHANICS,
with an Account of the Materials and Appliances used in Mechanical Dentistry, by OAKLEY COLES, L.D.S.R.C.S., Surgeon-Dentist to the Hospital for Diseases of the Throat. Second Edition, crown 8vo, with 140 Engravings, 7s. 6d. [1876]

HANDBOOK OF DENTAL ANATOMY
and Surgery for the use of Students and Practitioners by JOHN SMITH, M.D., F.R.S. Edin., Surgeon-Dentist to the Queen in Scotland. Second Edition, fcap 8vo, 4s. 6d. [1871]

STUDENT'S GUIDE TO DENTAL ANATOMY AND SURGERY,
by HENRY SEWILL, M.R.C.S., L.D.S., late Dentist to the West London Hospital. With 77 Engravings, fcap. 8vo, 5s. 6d. [1876]

OPERATIVE DENTISTRY:
A Practical Treatise, by JONATHAN TAFT, D.D.S., Professor of Operative Dentistry in the Ohio College of Dental Surgery. Third Edition, thoroughly revised, with many additions, and 134 Engravings, 8vo, 18s. [1877]

DENTAL CARIES
and its Causes: an Investigation into the influence of Fungi in the Destruction of the Teeth, by Drs. LEBER and ROTTENSTEIN. Translated by H. CHANDLER, D.M.D., Professor in the Dental School of Harvard University. With Illustrations, royal 8vo, 5s. [1878]

The following CATALOGUES issued by Messrs CHURCHILL will be forwarded post free on application:

1. *Messrs Churchill's General List of nearly* 600 *works on Medicine, Surgery, Midwifery, Materia Medica, Hygiene, Anatomy, Physiology, Chemistry, &c., &c., with a complete Index to their Titles, for easy reference.* N.B.—*This List includes Nos.* 2 *and* 3.

2. *Selection from Messrs Churchill's General List, comprising all recent Works published by them on the Art and Science of Medicine.*

3. *A selected and descriptive List of Messrs Churchill's Works on Chemistry, Materia Medica, Pharmacy, Botany, Photography, Zoology, the Microscope, and other branches of Science.*

4. *The Medical Intelligencer, an Annual List of New Works and New Editions published by Messrs J. & A. Churchill, together with Particulars of the Periodicals issued from their House.*

[Sent in January of each year to every Medical Practitioner in the United Kingdom whose name and address can be ascertained. A large number are also sent to the United States of America, Continental Europe, India, and the Colonies.]

MESSRS CHURCHILL have a special arrangement with MESSRS LINDSAY & BLAKISTON, OF PHILADELPHIA, in accordance with which that Firm act as their Agents for the United States of America, either keeping in Stock most of Messrs CHURCHILL's Books, or reprinting them on Terms advantageous to Authors. Many of the Works in this Catalogue may therefore be easily obtained in America.

PRINTED BY J. E. ADLARD, BARTHOLOMEW CLOSE.

www.ingramcontent.com/pod-product-compliance
Lightning Source LLC
Chambersburg PA
CBHW031833230426
43669CB00009B/1327